THE DYSLEXIC CHILD

Today we take it for granted that every child has some ability with language, and we consider children who have difficulty as being stupid or lazy. Yet in fact they may be suffering from dyslexia or word-blindness, a disability which has only recently become widely recognized and which, with proper help, may be improved.

Dyslexic children may confuse letters like b and d, and often reverse letters and words or leave part of the word out, and their spelling often has a characteristic bizarre quality. Although they may be very intelligent, their difficulties in reading and spelling may hold them back in school, and it is important that the condition should be recognized early and special remedial treatment begun at once so that the child can catch up in school and begin to enjoy reading.

Professor Miles shows how the conditions can be identified and how help can be given. This book is essential reading for parents, teachers and social workers, and will give much needed guidance to all who wish to understand the condition and help the sufferers.

The foreword is contributed by Oliver Zangwill, Professor of Experimental Psychology in the University of Cambridge and Consultant Psychologist to the National Hospital for Nervous Diseases, Queen Square, London, who has made a major contribution to the study of dyslexia.

PRIORY EDITORIAL CONSULTANTS

THE CARE AND WELFARE LIBRARY

Consultant Medical Editor: Alexander R. K. Mitchell,
MB, ch.B, MRCPE, MRCPsych.

THE
DYSLEXIC CHILD

T. R. MILES
MA, ph.D, FBPS.S

Professor of Psychology, University College of North Wales, Bangor

Foreword by

PROFESSOR OLIVER ZANGWILL

PRIORY PRESS LIMITED

The Care and Welfare Library

The Alcoholic and the Help He Needs Max Glatt, MD, FRCPsych., MRCP, DPM

Drugs—The Parents' Dilemma Alexander R. K. Mitchell, MB, ch.B, MRCPE, MRCPsych.

Schizophrenia Alexander R. K. Mitchell, MB, ch.B, MRCPE, MRCPsych.

Sex and the Love Relationship Faith Spicer, MB, BS, JP

V.D. Explained Roy Statham, MB, ch.B

The Care of the Aged Dennis Hyams, MB, FRCP

Aggression in Youth Roy Ridgway

Stress in Industry Joseph L. Kearns, MB, BCh., MSC.

The Child Under Stress Edna Oakeshott, Ph.D

Student Health Philip Cauthery, MB, ch.B, DPH

The Slow-to-Learn James Ellis, MEd.

I.Q.—150 Sydney Bridges, MA, MEd., Ph.D

When Father is Away The Rev. A. H. Denney, AKC, BA

Healing through Faith Christopher Woodard, MRCS, LRCP

Sexual Variations John Randell, MD, FRCP

Children in Hospital—The Parents' View Ann Hales-Tooke, MA

The Baby's First Days James Partridge, MA, MB, BCh.

Allergies Douglas Blair Macaulay, MD

Migraine Edda Hanington, MD

The Dyslexic Child T. R. Miles, MA, Ph.D, FBPS.S

Health in Middle Age Michael Green, MA, MB, BCh.

Care of the Dying Richard Lamerton, MRCS, LRCP

Depression—The Blue Plague A. H. Watts, OBE, MD

SBN 85078 096 9
Copyright © 1974 by T. R. Miles
First published in 1974 by
Priory Press Limited
101 Grays Inn Road London WC1
Made and printed in Great Britain by
The Garden City Press Limited
Letchworth, Hertfordshire SG6 1JS

Contents

Foreword

by O. L. Zangwill

AS every parent knows, children differ enormously in the facility with which they learn to read. While some seem to pick it up almost effortlessly, others, apparently no less intelligent, find it difficult and discouraging. Teachers, too, are very well aware of such differences, not only in learning to read but also in learning to spell which, for some slow readers at least, appears to present almost insurmountable difficulties. As a result, slow learners readily become sensitive and frustrated, especially when there are younger brothers or sisters already showing signs of outstripping them in school progress. Reading, therefore, must be regarded as a skill which by no means every child of normal intelligence can easily master, no matter how well and patiently taught. Moreover, some children —fortunately only a very small minority—find difficulties with reading and spelling out of all proportion to their intellectual competence and in spite of every encouragement they have received from parents and teachers. Why is this? And, perhaps even more important, what can we do about it?

These are the questions to which Professor T. R. Miles addresses himself in this lucid and sensible book. As he makes clear, the book is concerned not with backward

7

readers generally, but only with that relatively small proportion of them as may properly be called *dyslexic*, that is, those with severe reading problems which can be ascribed neither to overall lack of intelligence or educational opportunity nor to emotional or social difficulties at home or at school. As Professor Miles makes clear, these are children who, while in no sense physically or mentally abnormal, do in fact suffer from a genuine developmental handicap. Their disability is educational rather than medical in the ordinary sense.

This handicap was at one time known as "word-blindness" and it is significant that some of the earliest reports of it came from ophthalmologists, who had obviously been consulted by the parents of dyslexic children in the belief that they might conceivably have been suffering from an obscure disorder of visual recognition. Although this may indeed be so, in some cases at least, there can be no doubt that the source of the disability lies not in the eye but in the brain. In consequence, the disorder has come to be regarded as in some sense neurological, though it is evident that it need not be associated with any obvious signs of brain injury. As Professor Miles quite properly suggests, dyslexia may best be regarded as "constitutional," in so far as it is "built into" the bodily constitution either through inheritance or possibly through the vicissitudes of development in the earliest years of life.

For this reason, the condition is often known as *specific* or *developmental dyslexia*. It is *specific* in so far as it is independent of intelligence or memory in general (although there are often associated features) and it is *developmental* in so far as it bears upon the acquisition of reading and spelling skills rather than upon breakdown of these skills after they have been acquired, as may occur in an older child or adult in consequence of injury or disease of the brain. Unlike many forms of psychological difficulty which may have a bearing upon education, in particular the neuroses and behaviour disorders which are the province of the psychiatrist, developmental dyslexia depends only in very minor ways upon external or environmental factors—though this is not of course to say that it is entirely unaffected by environmental influence. Indeed, the goal of helping dyslexic children through the development of teaching methods especially directed towards the overcoming of their special difficulties is obviously that to which research should be directed and clearly animates the writer of this book.

The earliest explanation to be given of developmental dyslexia is that it might be due to maldevelopment of a small part of the brain which is thought to be concerned with the acquisition and control of reading. Although damage of the area in question is known to disrupt reading in the adult, there is no evidence of any structural brain disorder in developmental dyslexia, though some more subtle impairment or "lag" in its functional development may of course exist. It is unlikely, however, that the error can be traced to any very specifically localized mechanism (or what used to be called a "centre") in a particular part of the brain.

A second explanation was advanced by an American paediatric neurologist, S. T. Orton, who was perhaps the first medical man to appreciate the educational implications of clinical neurology. Orton was much struck by the incidence of left-handedness and mixed hand-preferences among dyslexic children, as also by the incidence of reversal errors in their writing, and even occasionally in their speech. For these he coined the unaesthetic neologism *strephosymbolia* (literally, "twisted symbols"). Strephosymbolia, which is of course common in the writing of young children, is shown in such errors as confusion of b with d or of p with q, and may involve reversal of the order of letters within a word, e.g. "saw" for "was." But whereas such errors are soon eliminated by normal readers, they may persist for some years among dyslexic children and are eliminated only with much difficulty. Orton believed that these errors arise in consequence of competition between the two cerebral hemispheres in the control of reading and spelling, which he attributed to the lack of firm lateral preferences and in consequence to the failure of one hemisphere to achieve the normal exclusive control of language and speech. This hemisphere, normally the left, has long been known as the dominant hemisphere, and dyslexia could thus be ascribed to a failure to establish normal cerebral dominance.

Although Orton's theory is in many ways attractive, it is, admittedly, very speculative. While left and mixed-handedness do occur very frequently in dyslexic children and their families, most left or mixed handed children learn to read normally and further factors must undoubtedly play a part. Furthermore, recent work has cast some doubt on the relation between handedness and cerebral dominance, and it now seems plain that the dominant hemisphere in most partly or even wholly left-handed individuals is the left, and not the right as was long supposed. Nonetheless, there is at the least a strong possibility that difficulty in learning to read and spell is linked in some way with the issue of cerebral dominance, though exactly what this relation is has still to be ascertained.

A third explanation—and the one most popular today —is that dyslexia results from a retardation in the general development of language ("developmental lag") and that this handicap tends to run in families, in other words, its basis is genetical. Reading and spelling are acquired later and with greater voluntary effort than the acquisition of spoken language, and are accordingly more severely affected by this developmental handicap. As we now know, many (though not all) dyslexic children turn out to have been relatively slow in learning to talk, and as Professor Miles indicates, some residual difficulty in articulation or sentence structure may be apparent much later on, especially if it is looked for. Further, there is often residual difficulty in what one might call "high-level" verbal activity, for example in written composition, in precis-writing, or on undertaking those tasks which psychologists refer to as "verbal" intelligence tests. This need imply no general want of intelligence, merely a limitation in the intellectual uses and applications of language.

At the same time, the evidence for a genetical basis is still largely circumstantial. As Professor Miles points out, it is suggested by the frequent incidence of language retardation or reading difficulty in the family history of dyslexic children, by the far higher incidence of dyslexia in boys than in girls, suggesting a partially sex-linked factor, and perhaps by the not infrequent association of dyslexia with familial left-handedness, particularly, perhaps, in the mother. Unfortunately, the geneticists can still tell us nothing very precise about the inheritance either of left-handedness or of learning disability; in fact the position is just about as obscure as in the vexed problem of the inheritance of intellectual capacity.

It is still widely supposed that if the origin of a disorder, physical or mental, is "genetical," that is inherited, nothing whatsoever can be done to alleviate it. Indeed theories of mental disorder based on the concept of an inherited predisposition are often dubbed fatalistic, the implication being that no treatment is possible. Nothing could be further from the truth. In our own time, we have seen one variety of educational subnormality (phenylketonuria) virtually eliminated by early diagnosis and correction through dietary means of an inborn error of metabolism. We have seen, too, much serious psychiatric illness which depends, at least in part, on genetical predisposition greatly relieved, and sometimes indeed apparently cured, by medication and environmental modification. In the same way, the fact that dyslexia has a constitutional foundation provides no reason whatsoever to relax remedial effort: it merely redoubles the need for it.

Although I have spoken of dyslexia as "specific," this does not mean that it may not be associated with other features, which may or may not contribute to the central difficulties in reading and spelling. Indeed Professor Miles specifies a number of things, among them a tendency to confuse left and right; poor immediate memory for words, letters or digits—a factor which almost certainly contributes to the spelling difficulty; troubles in learning and reciting arithmetical tables and sometimes, too, a curious difficulty in retaining order of sequence which may lead, for example, to using the correct letters in spelling a word but putting them in the wrong order. The extent to which these various difficulties are cause or effect of the basic trouble in reading and spelling has still to be determined. At all events, dyslexia—to use a medical term—is better described as a "syndrome," that is as a constellation of associated difficulties, rather than as a difficulty in reading and spelling in the narrow sense.

Although Professor Miles does not enter into detail about methods of remedial education, his short account of the problem of seeking remedial help and its implications for parents will be of great value. As in so many fields in which a disability, though only too obvious to those affected and to those around them, has yet to be fully recognized at an administrative level, dyslexia poses a most difficult problem for parents as well as for those teachers who have become aware of its incidence and nature. His shrewd account will be found useful by many, particularly by baffled parents seeking help and advice in an educational world still largely uncomprehending of their child's handicap. One hopes that this book will be widely read and that its message will gradually filter through to all concerned with making the best of our educational potential in the challenging world of today.

Psychological Laboratory
University of Cambridge, 1974

I

Four Case Studies

THIS book is addressed to parents, doctors, teachers, administrators, psychologists, social workers, and indeed to anyone else who wishes to find out more about dyslexia. I shall introduce the subject by citing four case studies, all of which seem to me to illustrate forcibly the difficulties experienced by dyslexic children. Chapters 2 and 3 are concerned with diagnosis and Chapter 4 with causation. After that I discuss problems of screening in Chapter 5, problems of morale in Chapter 6 and problems of organizing suitable teaching in Chapter 7. Finally, in Chapter 8, I cite some further case studies designed to illustrate the prospects for a dyslexic child as he grows up.

I shall not make any detailed suggestions with regard to teaching procedures since I have done this elsewhere (see Further Reading, p. 136, nos. 11 and 12). Rather, my main purpose will be to show how dyslexic children can be recognized and how provision can be made, both at school and in the home, for helping them.

No attempt will be made at detailed documentation of the views which I shall put forward, though confirmatory evidence is available in most of the references given on pp. 135–6. Any book of this kind must of necessity be based in some measure on the writer's personal experience, but I have tried not to depart in any serious way from the consensus among those who take the concept of dyslexia seriously.

No two cases of dyslexia are exactly alike. Indeed, in view of the many kinds of variation which exist in nature this is not surprising. Once one has seen a few cases, however, there emerges a clear basic pattern. Its essential features are: difficulty over learning to spell despite adequate opportunity and intelligence, difficulty over learning to read, difficulty in some tasks involving awareness of left and right, difficulty over arranging things in the correct temporal sequence, difficulty with certain kinds of items involving short-term memory, and sometimes difficulty over subtraction and difficulty in learning and reciting arithmetical tables. In the case of any particular skill a dyslexic child can learn to compensate for some of these difficulties; as a result of hard effort, for instance, he will probably become able to read more or less adequately, and even spelling may eventually not be too much of a problem. One is left in no doubt, however, that such a child has a handicap, and to judge his performance by standards appropriate to those without this handicap is bound to create unhappiness.

The four people whom I shall describe in this chapter— Henry aged 10, John and Laura both aged 15, and Robert aged 19—can, I think, be regarded as typical cases of dyslexia in almost all respects. Admittedly it is possible to be less severely handicapped than they were, and the handicap can be less crippling when special teaching is arranged at an earlier age, preferably by the time the child is aged 8. Between them, however, these four cases seem to me to provide a clear illustration of the problems which a dyslexic child is likely to meet in the present educational system, particularly if his dyslexia is not recognized by his teachers.

The information which I shall be presenting is based on the correspondence in my files and on the notes which I made at the time. I have changed the four names, but otherwise I have tried to record what happened as accurately as possible.

Case 1: Henry

Henry's father was a doctor, who wrote to me as follows:

"Our son aged 10 suffers from this disability [sc. dyslexia] though I have not been able to get anyone within the Educational Authority in which we live to accept him as a dyslexic and this is causing me considerable unhappiness and concern ... Without an authoritative assessment of my son, it has proved extremely difficult for me to bring any influence to bear on the County Department of Education in terms of getting any recognition of a disability in my child. In fact it has been suggested to me that he is just educationally backward, though one assessment ... left me wondering whether —— had any realization of the occurrence of dyslexia, let alone any understanding of it."

I first saw Henry when he was aged 10½. I gave him some of the tests described in Chapter 2, and found him

• •

to be well above average in general reasoning power. I am hesitant to quote I.Q. figures since there are all kinds of pitfalls and possibilities of misunderstanding, but, for what it is worth, his I.Q. on the Terman test (see p. 55) came out at 123 (where average is 100 and only $2\frac{1}{2}$ per cent of the population are expected to score over 130). In contrast, when I gave him tests of reading and spelling his performance was approximately that of an 8-year old. This discrepancy between intellectual level and performance at reading and spelling was clearly something which needed to be taken seriously.

I noticed regular confusion between b and d, although almost all children of normal ability grow out of such confusion by age 8 at the latest: he read "big" for "dig" and when given the word "dream" he started with a b-sound also when given the word "biscuit" he started with a d-sound. In a piece of written work "bide" had been put for "died" and "umber" had been written for "under." He himself spontaneously said, "I sometimes get b and d back to front." He also read "was" instead of "saw" and wrote "on" for "no."

He had difficulty in repeating the polysyllabic words "preliminary," "anemone," and "statistical." He showed signs of losing his place in reciting the seven times table and omitted "October" in reciting the months of the year. When given three digits and asked to say them backwards he failed on one of the two occasions. These are all items on which those with dyslexia have been found to experience difficulty.

The following are some samples of his spelling taken from school books:

17

"There are meny strange and fasen(t crossed out)ating fisf, but it seems difecolt to belever that some fish are kapabul of generating ther (crossings out) whone ELEstricaty wh (crossed out) with which they can guve (?) a shoc ... these fish have an orgen behind eash (changed to each) ire which is a mase of sels, roth like a a hone kome."

("There are many strange and fascinating fish, but it seems difficult to believe that some fish are capable of generating their own electricity with which they can give a shock ... These fish have an organ behind each ear which is a mass of cells, rather like a honeycomb.")

"There whars on anser to this ecsept the noding of a fyuw heads and the ciking of the smallest sistes a ganst the tadule. And of curs it wars truw, the chulgren war thin and poor and they never had enuf to eat. The onie father had bide in a storm a foue years Be for."

("There was no answer to this except the nodding of a few heads and the kicking of the smallest sister's [foot] against the table. And of course it was true. The children were thin and poor and they never had enough to eat. Their own father had died in a storm a few years before.")

A dyslexic child will often spell a word in several different ways on successive occasions: Henry's inconsistencies over "fish" and "few" are examples. Also syllables may be omitted or put in the wrong order, as in "elestricaty" for "electricity." Sometimes losing the place

There are meny strange and fasenting fish, but it seems defecolt to belever that some fish are Kapabul of generating thett ~~the other~~ Whone ELEstricaty ~~totte~~ with Which they can gule a shoc

the best none of these fish live in whorm seas these fish have an orger behind each in which is a mase of sels. roth like a a Kone Kome

There Whars on anser to this ecsept the noding of a fyuw heads and the ciKing of the Smallest sistes a gunst the tadule. And of curs it Wars truW.

the chulgren Wer thin and poor and they never had enuf to eat. The one father had Hide in a storm a foue years Be for

Writing by a dyslexic boy aged 10.

takes the form of repeating a word or syllable, as in the repetition of the word "a" in the first passage; and sometimes there seems to be no clear sense of where one word ends and another one begins, as in "a ganst" for "against" and "Be for" for "before". It is these kinds of errors, as well as the b-d confusion, which often give the spelling of dyslexic children its bizarre character.

It is, however, highly intelligent spelling. Given that one cannot remember how a word is spelled, one can still sometimes *deduce* the correct spelling by sounding the parts of the word to oneself, and this is in fact what Henry appears to have been doing. Even when the spelling is totally wrong, as in "fyuw" for "few," it is often possible to see the logic behind it; and from the phonetic point of view many of his attempts, even when wrong, are remarkably accurate.

I had no hesitation in confirming with Henry's parents that he was dyslexic. Later sections of this book will indicate in more detail what this implies, but, briefly, to use the word "dyslexic" is to say that the difficulties are constitutional in origin, or, in other words, that there is some failure (though we do not know the details) in the mechanisms for perception and memory. This means that one cannot regard such things as poor teaching or parental anxiety as primary causal factors. It also means that the person has a disability—a definite *handicap*—which needs to be compensated for; and experience shows that special teaching on an individual basis is essential if he is to be helped.

The word "dyslexia," when used of a boy such as Henry, seems to me to have three main functions: it classifies, it explains, and it invites to action. It classifies in that it distinguishes those who display this group of difficulties from those who do not, and the claim is that the difference is important; it explains in that it points out that the difficulties are constitutional in origin, and it invites to action in that, once a child has been classified as dyslexic, this implies the need for special teaching techniques.

The first thing, as far as Henry and his parents were concerned, was to give them a clear account of what the difficulties were. This I tried to do. Clearly it is no use offering remedies until one knows what is wrong. On the other hand it is a widely accepted maxim that diagnosis without treatment is unethical, and in Henry's neighbourhood there seemed to be no one who even knew about dyslexia, let alone had the necessary skills for teaching him. In this particular case we arranged that both Henry and his mother should come to me together for a "crash course" lasting a week and that his mother should take over the teaching from there. During this week I tried to show her the basic principles, as I understood them, that were needed for the teaching of any dyslexic child. One of the first requirements, of course, was to try to give Henry confidence; but this could not be done merely by telling him that he was an able boy. What was needed was to give him a taste of success; and I tried to show his mother how to move to progressively more difficult spelling tasks while making sure that each stage was properly learned before he went on to the next one. I shall not attempt to go into details here, but, briefly, the methods used were those described by Miss G. C. Cotterell (see Further Reading, p. 135, reference 2, Chapter 8, pp. 49–70), and by myself (see p. 136, reference 11); and it was not difficult to pass them on to Henry's mother. I do not wish to give the impression that parental coaching is the answer in *all* cases of dyslexia; some parents may not feel competent to make the attempt, and in some cases other facilities may be available. It is, however, a possibility which should certainly be given serious consideration.

Case 2: John

I first saw John at the age of 15. One of the things which I was shown was a poem which he had written at the age of 10, for which he had been awarded a prize in a competition.* I shall quote this poem in full—not as an illustration of his spelling (since the version which I saw had presumably been edited) but simply to indicate some of his feelings. The poem was entitled *What punishment is next?* and it went as follows:

"I am tortured every day
My hands or feet are blown away
A rook's nest in my head, feathers in my shirt
Handed down from farmers' wives.
What punishment is next?

"I am lonely and the birds won't come near me
Unless to take a grain of straw.

* I am grateful to the Editor of the *Dyslexia Review*, Mrs. V. W. Fisher, for permission to reprint this poem.

But me—I am hung on a frame
And cannot fight the evil world.

"When gale force winds whistle past my ear—
That will be my dying day.
Me, a scarecrow, dead, nothing left.
No punishment is left."

The following information was given to me by John's mother in a letter: "John's first three years at school (local state) were very unhappy and he was placed in a backward class in the Junior School. He was behind with his reading but his biggest difficulty was his writing. After several abortive attempts to produce something that was suitably legible to gain his teachers' approval he almost gave up trying. The small amount of work he produced was mirror writing. He found it impossible to distinguish b from d, and some of his numbers were back to front [She drew a reversed 5 and a reversed 7.] Sometimes his answers were reversed, e.g. $5 \times 3 = 51$. We took him to see the educational psychologist and then subsequently were sent to see —— the psychiatrist ... Briefly, he was an intelligent child with problems. We were advised to send him to a small private school. After an uphill struggle he managed to write but it was very illegible and dreadful spelling. Being able to write seemed to release a lot of tension and he began to write poetry. [He] returned to a state school at the age of thirteen years. He has learned to improvise ways to overcome some of his difficulties. He uses capital letters sometimes in preference to small letters because he does not have to worry about which way they face. Over the past two years he has tried very hard to improve the legibility of his handwriting with considerable success but his erratic spelling persists. Sometimes his words are quite correct but sometimes he will use two separate spellings for the same word in the one sentence, speak, speeck ... Sometimes he will add extra letters, post, poast. His creative writing is considered very good and he has a love of language, but we have been told that he will not get 'O' level English if he does not master the basic skills, i.e. spelling, punctuation. It has been suggested he could do quite well at physics if he could write more straightforward notes ... Although he is now a much happier child, I think sometimes at school he feels demoralized."

She also sent a school report. Among other comments it contained the following:

"English:

A hardworking boy with a maturity of outlook and ideas but who cannot express these ideas in writing, which is undisciplined with frequent misspellings and missing full stops. His handwriting also is badly formed.

"History:

A conscientious boy who finds difficulty in expressing himself on paper. His writing is often illegible although verbally he is quite mature. Probably an average C.S.E. prospect.

"Spanish:

>An excellent pupil in all but one respect—he finds difficulty in writing correct Spanish. However, there have been definite signs of improvement and I am quite confident that with encouragement he will overcome this weakness.

"Geography:

>He gives the impression that he is hardworking but very often this is an illusion. He needs continual supervision of homework and classwork. It should be pointed out, however, that he is always pleasant and helpful.

"French:

>John is a hardworking boy, who copes well with oral French but he cannot transfer this knowledge correctly onto paper. In the examination his performance was poor due to this difficulty, and it would seem that his chances of passing 'O' level next year will be marred.

"Physics:

>Works hard. Exam result this time shows the definate [sic] improvement I have been hoping for."

Before presenting my own findings, I should like to call attention to a number of points in the letter from John's mother and in his school report. I will begin with the former.

First, it seems that a highly intelligent boy had been placed in a backward class and was very unhappy there. Second, the discouragement was such that he "almost gave up trying." Third, the boy tended to do figures the wrong way round and to confuse b and d. Fourth, he had learned ways of compensating for his disability. Fifth, the same word might be spelled differently even in the same sentence. The difficulties reported here seemed to me clearly to be those of someone with dyslexia, and the early unhappiness is, regrettably, all too frequent.

I find it hard to comment fairly on the school report. No one, I am sure, could claim that there is anything really vicious or hostile in it, but I think one can fairly say that there is lack of imagination and lack of understanding. The "maturity of outlook" reported by the English master is in interesting contrast with his "frequent misspellings;" he is reported as "conscientious" at history, "always pleasant and helpful" in geography, and "hardworking" at French and physics. Yet he is "probably an average C.S.E. prospect" and the impression that he is hardworking is "very often . . . an illusion." Also his exam result in mathematics "did not reflect his true ability" and his chances of passing "O" level French will be "marred" by his weakness at written work. I have known other dyslexic children who were in fact very bright but who, because of their difficulties, were reckoned by their teachers to be "average." If one reads between the lines, one can imagine the kind of struggle which John was having at school. The incongruities are plain: he is mature yet only an average C.S.E. prospect; he is good orally but cannot get things down on paper; he has the standards in French and mathematics but cannot cope with traditional written examinations. Clearly he was right out of place in the "backward class" at his first school, yet progress in academic courses is held back because of his difficulty in passing examinations. The pressures which our educational system brings to bear on a dyslexic child can sometimes, I am sure, be quite bewildering. Indeed it is perhaps surprising that most dyslexic children survive these pressures as well as they do.

John's mother told me that an earlier testing had given an I.Q. of 132, which is, of course, a very high figure. I myself gave him a difficult reasoning test and he scored higher than the average specified for grammar school boys of his age, which scarcely squares with his being "an average C.S.E. prospect," but when asked to read words out of context he was by no means free of error, and when given a standard spelling test he made an appreciable number of mistakes.

Some pages from his history book are reproduced on pp.28–9. Elsewhere in his written work I noticed, among others, the following misspellings: "marie on Twanet" for "Marie Antoinette" (later written as "marie anne twanete"), "woemen" for "women," "pniced" for "panicked" (later written as "panniced"), "indenoty" for "indemnity," "treay, for "treaty," "dission" for "decision," and "candediture" for "candidature."

When asked to show his right hand he said, "I have

british Suez canal and would porosly annex the british market thus this met she was in favor of keeping the balkans as ssprte states so as russia could not move through them into the Mediterranean which Britons aside is so her personal party balke then there was Austria Hungary she wanted to annexs the balkas as her territorial ambition but If russia got in before her she could not root russia out so she had to be content with second best ie keeping russia out of the balkans thus if Austria Hungary was indeed compay told to as a matter of course france had interest in south africa as did not want them disturbed by russia ond so she sided with the morarity in keeping russia out but russia did not expect the other pores to join in after her war with Tenney a trey was signed the treaty of San stefano in which turkey had to promise to give the states of th balkas liberty thus the other powers combined to keep russia out at the congress of Berlin at which Bismark sat as Honest Broke thus the other powers stopped russia the honor and ruthlessness in the balkans is illustrated by the case of the war the two hundred christins in Armenia were living in savator and thus they decided to march into constantiople and take the palace this they did, immediatly the king ordered a troop of irregular guards to put down the rebellion and 2000 armeins lost their lives through the ruthless slaghter of a guerillos aid

28

later on however there was a complete arises of
the situation when easter rumelia rebelled and
joined Bulgaria thus the Anti russian feeling
of easter rumelia spread into Bulgia thus russia
thought she could deal with them one at a time but
note both together thus she tried to seperate
them thus the other powers ~~joined~~ act told
russia to leave the ~~two~~ powers alone the states
of Serbia, Herthzagovina, eastern rumelia and
Bulgaria discided to join togther to drive
as a united Balkan legues turkey out of
europe this they succeded in doing but at the
trety of potsmouth ~~rachpshlive~~ it was shown
that the other powers had different ideas
as to how the states were split up this
also went to slow the increasing importance
of America in european History

*   this cadediture was known as the LoenBoller
candiditure

I find it virtually impossible to read your
writing.

to think which one I write with," and when I asked which was *my* right hand (I was sitting opposite him), he turned round in his seat, saying "Let's think" and finally came up with the correct answer. In explanation he said, "I was going to that one [my left hand] as this is my right. But you are sitting opposite so I changed my mind." When asked to say "5-7-4" backwards he said "4-5-7" and when asked to say "2-5-9" backwards he said "5-9-2." He was, however, able to repeat various polysyllabic words, for example "preliminary" and "statistical," after me with no error. I gathered from his explanation that this was a skill which he had acquired through practice. His comment was: "I do a lot of this in Spanish; when two words are similar you've got to pick out the differences."

His mother also reported that he had no sense of time: thus he might dress and say he was going along to the shops even though it was late in the evening or a Sunday afternoon.

When I spoke to him informally I was fascinated by his account of his difficulties. Here are some extracts from the notes which I made at the time: "If I am in a sombre mood I write about infinity. They write about football ... Just my punctuation and spelling hold me back ... I've suddenly started to spell Spanish properly ... Sometimes when I'm writing an exam—say composition in English—I have to stop; its like a mental block; it's for a few seconds. I don't know what it is. It gets you annoyed. Possibly something to do with my subconscious—I'm checking the line above.

"I used to have difficulty with reading and writing.

Spelling difficulty didn't become apparent until I'd cleaned the writing up. Mother was very good—she bought me some books" [Q. Do you read for pleasure?] "Some books maintain my interest—Lorenz on aggression —fish, ducks—I found it very interesting. I am interested in computers . . . Alistair Mclean, John Wyndham, *Coral Island*—I suddenly realized I'd read two hundred pages and that it wasn't particularly hard going. Reading comes more quickly than writing . . . sometimes I just wanted to go out and play golf . . . but will-power. I can write legibly now except when I am in a hurry. I am poor on punctuation but it's beginning to come . . . very few full stops—there's a lull and you put a full stop . . . I had to scrawl it down the best I could.

"I'm fascinated by physics. Also psychology—there was a fascinating programme on movement; do you need biology? I don't like cutting up animals . . . I can never remember 7×8—mental block almost; I can do it when I think about it. The nine times I never bothered to learn. Just multiply by ten and take the number away . . . I've suddenly started to spell Spanish properly, not French."

I have met few dyslexic children who were able to be so articulate about their difficulties. The basic facts were plain: he was an intelligent boy who had had special difficulty with reading and spelling; he had many of the associated signs of dyslexia, viz. bizarre spelling, b-d confusion, difficulty in tasks involving appreciation of left and right, difficulty in repeating digits reversed, and difficulty in remembering multiplication tables. As will be pointed out in Chapter 2, it is the occurrence of this cluster of difficulties which entitles one to say that a person is dyslexic, with all that this implies. The reported lack of sense of time seems undoubtedly to be part of the same picture. Spanish was probably easier for him to spell than French because of its phonetic regularity.

Because John lived at a distance and in any case was over the worst as regards reading and spelling, I did not attempt to arrange any special tuition. I was able, however, in a written report, to make a number of recommendations, for example, that he should be given extra time in his examinations; this seemed to me particularly necessary in mathematics, where rechecking of computations was bound to take an extra long time. I indicated that his potential ability at mathematics might not show up if he was continually tied down with problems of computation, and that in many subjects, especially French, he would be likely to fare much better if he was examined orally. The examination system is plainly not geared, at present, to the needs of those such as John, and there seems to me a strong case for pressing for appropriate changes. Meanwhile it was possible for me to discuss the situation with John and his parents and give suitable encouragement, while making clear that I appreciated his difficulties and his efforts to overcome them.

Case 3: Laura

Two years ago I received a letter from a speech therapist about a girl aged 15. It said "I feel that Laura needs specialized help ... She is better at practical work than at academic and I am sure that her lack of ability to spell has hampered her progress in many respects, not the least being a severe lack of confidence when asked to write anything down ... Attempts to provide a teacher who could help Laura on a tutorial basis have, so far, failed as there is a shortage in this area of suitable personnel."

The speech therapist had in fact gone to enormous trouble to find help for Laura. Alas! It was a case of bureaucracy at its worst—so much so that I was moved to make a record of the correspondence which had been written about Laura during the nineteen months before I saw her.

17th Sept. (Letter from neurologist to G.P.) "There is no dyslexia. Mime is perfectly understood."

29th Sept. (Letter from hospital speech therapist to Laura's mother) "I ... find she is of school age. I regret that I am unable to see her as the county speech therapist undertakes all such cases. May I suggest you refer her to ..."

Undated (Letter from County Medical Officer to Laura's mother): "On making enquiries it has been found that Laura does not attend a L.E.A. school and therefore does not come within the provisions made by the ——shire Education Committee ... I was wondering whether it would be better to make arrangements with the Hospital Speech Therapist."

28th Oct. (Letter from neurologist to speech therapist) "I am a little bit annoyed about it [the above letter]."

12th Dec. (Psychologist's report) "A very pleasant but anxious and tense girl ... Laura's spelling is not a particular difficulty ... Laura has been advized to write out her spelling mistakes very many times, so that she has a chance of substituting the motor movement for the visual appearance of the work."

Jan. (undated) (Headmistress's report): "She is below average ability . . . she appears brighter than she actually is and has never mastered the art of spelling."

13th April (Letter from speech therapist to Laura's mother): "We are still working at obtaining help for Laura with her reading etc. . . . I . . . hope you can be patient a little longer."

19th May (Letter from Group Secretary to Laura's mother): "I am sorry for the delay in starting Laura's tuition."

Spring (No exact date). (From speech therapist's notes) "The teacher employed by the hospital said she would undertake the duties, then changed her mind."

Summer (as above). "An excellent teacher who has retired was employed by the hospital (after much discussion in the —— office who said it was creating a precedent to employ a *teacher* for *treatment*). Dr. Y [the neurologist] backed me on every occasion."

August (as above). "Mother admitted for surgery . . . Disruption in the family caused teacher to be irritated by lack of communication. Teaching programme abandoned by teacher—much to mother's dismay."

Autumn (as above). "A deputy head teacher of good ability [was] employed by the hospital to teach Laura twice a week. This teacher was suddenly promoted to Acting Headmistress of another school and felt she could not undertake Laura's programme."

15th Jan. (Letter from speech therapist to neurologist): "A seemingly impossible series of incidents have pre-

vented Laura from receiving treatment for dyslexia . . .
I should like to suggest she be referred to Dr. X . . ."

11th Mar. (Letter from Dr. X's secretary to the neurologist) "Dr. X has now retired from the N.H.S. . . . He is
still in private practice."

One week later I received the letter from the speech
therapist from which I have quoted above. I learned then
that Laura's mother was divorced and had recently needed
some intensive surgical treatment. I also learned that
Laura's headmistress had proposed to enter her for a
C.S.E. secretarial course!

I find this a dramatic case in that it illustrates both
human dedication and human failings. I was left with a
feeling of deep gratitude that there were such people as
the speech therapist, who had persevered in trying to
arrange help for Laura despite all kinds of setbacks. I
was also left with a feeling of dismay, not only at the
workings of bureaucracy, but at the fact that well-inten-
tioned people (as I am sure both the headmistress and the
psychologist were) should get things so hopelessly wrong!
To judge from the intelligence test results (see below) it
was simply not true that Laura was "below average
ability." She was dyslexic, however, and I can think of
few more unsuitable jobs for a dyslexic girl than secretarial ones. The psychologist's failure to mention dyslexia,
though not unexpected, was disappointing. The recom-
mendation that corrected spellings should be written out
many times was, I am almost sure, a useless one which
would have resulted only in increasing frustration, while
talk of "substituting the motor movement for the visual

appearance of the word" is, I suspect, pretentious nonsense.

My own testing showed Laura to be marginally above average in general reasoning ability, but she was below the 12-year level in reading and below the 11-year level in spelling. She had difficulty in responding correctly to questions such as "Point to my right ear with your left hand," in repeating polysyllabic words, in saying digits backwards, and in remembering arithmetical tables. Her mother reported that Laura had earlier had difficulty over b and d, and Laura herself said, "It's spelling I find most difficult. I tend to spell some things back to front." In her school books there were the following mistakes: "hoil-days," for "holidays," "solidrs" for "soldiers," "crital" for "critical," "strecaches" for "stretches," "amoinear" for "ammonia," "nessary" for "necessary," and "proect" for "protect." Her teacher had reported that she "will make mistakes which have been correctly written in previous exercises."

Laura was not an easy person to teach, and because of distance she could come to Bangor only once a week; but, despite complications due to her mother's illnesses, she persevered with one of the Bangor teachers for over a year, and when finally she decided to stop coming she wrote an extremely appreciative letter.

Case 4: Robert

Robert came to see me at the age of 19. His mother had written as follows: "Our local Child Guidance Clinic 'did not believe in making a diagnosis of dyslexia,' so, although he seemed a text book case, he never had an official diagnosis.

"He has done very well in overcoming his difficulty. He can read his text books, though he does not read for pleasure; and can write, though his spelling is still very uncertain. In spite of this he has four 'O' levels (Physics, Chemistry, Maths and Technical Drawing) and is at present studying for three 'A' level exams (Pure Maths, Applied Maths, and Physics). The difficulty lies in his inability to take English 'O' level ... He needs either to get this exam or to get exemption from it on the grounds of his disability ... I realize that it is much more difficult to make a firm assessment in the case of someone his age than for a boy of ten or eleven, but I think he presents an uncomplicated enough picture for the signs still to be clear."

I was able, without hesitation, to confirm that Robert was dyslexic. His reading still showed inaccuracies; for example presented with "siege" he said "sage, no siege," and presented with "pneumonia" he said "phenomenal, no pneumonia." Spelling mistakes were still common, and on one sheet I saw that he had actually misspelled his own name, writing "Rbert" for "Robert" (this was not his actual name but the mistake was similar). He was able to indicate the right and left sides of my body as I sat opposite him but only after considerable effort. He said that when he drove a car he found the instructions "turn right" and "turn left" very baffling. He failed to repeat the polysyllabic words "preliminary," "anemone," and "statistical" correctly and he lost his place in saying his seven-times table. I noticed that when I gave him particular test items he often had to ask for the instructions to be repeated, and his mother confirmed that people always "had to say it over again" for him.

I had already met two relatives of Robert's, an uncle and cousin, both of whom were dyslexic, and Robert's mother told me that some other relatives were also affected. (More details about the incidence of dyslexia in this family are given in Chapter 4.) The fact that other members of a family also have similar difficulties is, of course, itself confirmatory evidence of dyslexia in a particular case.

She also indicated the extent to which Robert had suffered earlier in life. I thought it would be interesting if she could supply me with further details, and a few weeks later she sent me a large amount of information, from which I have extracted the following: "... You must realize that an open invitation to a parent to ramble on about her child is liable to produce several volumes of closely written waffle! I can only say that I *have* tried to pick out the significant bits ...

"He was very slow in learning to talk and did not really start until he was two ... He started school very happily and settled down well. The only outstanding feature I can remember at this time is that he would periodically get very frustrated at some communication failure. After a series of these he would get very upset and have a long fit of crying ... After he had been at school for a bit I began to be concerned about his work. My brother had had difficulties in learning to read, and there were things about Robert which made me think he would have similar difficulties ...

"I asked for an intelligence test so that we could have

some sort of guide as to what progress it might be reasonable to expect. We did not want to worry if his slow progress was due to low intelligence. Of course, I was discouraged. 'Once you get into the hands of psychologists,' said the school doctor, 'you never know what will happen.' However, eventually two I.Q. tests were done. On the first . . . he scored an I.Q. of 120 and on the second 118.

"Shortly after this we moved and he changed schools. The new school was overfull and he was put straight into the junior section although he should really have had another term in the infants school. The school was streamed and he was soon transferred to the 'C' stream. From then on we heard very little about what was happening at school. We sometimes heard stories about one of the other children, but never anything about the classroom work. We wanted to give him time to settle so refrained from being too inquisitive. He seemed to like the teacher, and she would respond to enquiries by saying that he was very helpful in class, that he was a co-operative child, and so on.

"His behaviour at home deteriorated. He presented a classic picture of an unhappy child. He would come home and start to tease the dog, upset his younger brother, complain that his older brother had hit him, moon around not knowing what to do, sit down to watch T.V. and almost at once find he couldn't have the chair or the programme he wanted . . . or something else would be wrong. During the holidays he was different. Of course there were still arguments, but these were of the ordinary sort which can be settled by the children themselves. They made camps in the garden, had a rope to swing on from one of the trees, and made all sorts of things from old grocery boxes. It took some days at the beginning of the holidays for him to shake off the effects of the school term, and, as the holiday drew towards its end he started to slip back out of his 'holiday mood.' As he got older it took longer and longer for the effects of school to wear off, and he started to anticipate the end of the holidays earlier and earlier. By the time he was ten the Christmas and Easter holidays were too short for recovery. It was the reappearance of his old happy self for a few weeks during the long Summer holidays when he was ten (a self we had not seen for a year) that finally decided us that drastic action was needed. We felt that even the summer break might be too short next year.

"Of course we had been trying to do something for some time before this. When it was clear he was making very little progress at school we had seen his teachers who had all been as helpful as possible. We had been to the local Child Guidance Clinic and had had a battery of tests and interviews. The Educational Psychologist had estimated his I.Q. at 108 saying that the earlier assessment was 'an over optimistic forecast due to his age' but had agreed that his school work was far behind what he ought to be able to achieve. The psychologist said that he had done his best to find out if home circumstances, or my handling of him was causing his difficulties but had been unable to do so. He said that Robert was exceptionally introverted (something that anyone who saw him for more than a few minutes at this time could have seen) and that this was probably the cause of his difficulty. He would never be able to learn in the presence of other children.

"I disagreed. I thought the introversion was being caused by the learning difficulties rather than the other way round, and hoped that he would improve if he could learn to read. I set about trying to teach him myself, keeping him at home on every excuse I could invent while doing some reading and writing with him. I did not officially tell the teacher what I was doing as I did not want to put her in a false position, but I think she knew. She was very helpful, and lent us books and cards he was using at school. We did manage to help him a bit in this way but it was an uphill struggle. The methods I was using were different to those used by the school (no good using the methods by which he had already failed to learn) and every time he went back for a few days he lost most of the ground he had gained. However, by ten he was able to struggle through fairly simple material.

"His difficulty extended to arithmetic. He couldn't remember the order of numbers, confusing 12 and 21. The signs were also mixed. To him × and + looked the same. In a subtraction sum he could not remember which number he was taking from which, sometimes changing direction in the middle of a sum. Of course all these sums were marked wrong even though the actual calculations were right. This further confused him and he lost confidence in his skills at calculation. He thus got the idea that he was no good at maths and this conviction has taken years to grow out of. In fact I had always thought that he might be much better at maths than he thought. Many times when discussing a problem with his older brother, Robert would suddenly come out with the right answer, having seen the way to do the problem quickly . . . but the moment the problem was labelled 'maths' he dried up again.

"We had cast round for something he could do which would be his 'own thing.' He took up shell collecting with the help of a very nice neighbour who helped him classify them. In time he got quite a large collection. When asked why he was interested he said he liked the feel of them, and demonstrated this by running his fingers over the smooth interior of a mussel.

"Feeling that the thing he needed above all was to be removed from the pressure of having to attend classes, we sent him to the one school in England where this is possible. We had already looked round the local schools and had visited the local —— school. But the doctor who examined children before admission said that he thought Robert had some sort of disease of the nerves (possibly chorea) and refused him admission. This will give some idea of the state he was in at that time.

"Once he was removed from the pressures associated with school he started to grow up. We had always known he was 'young for his age.' What we had not realized was that he had stopped developing emotionally shortly after starting school. Once he was free to grow he developed emotionally at the rate of about one year per term. It took him about three years to catch up with his chronological age.

"It was some years before he wanted to do anything about his reading and writing.

"At the new school he went to pottery and art classes ... Finally he found out what interested him. He learned to play first the washboard, then drums and guitar in the school jazz band. He also showed an interest in electronics, and, one holiday, I read through a Tutor text book with him on the subject. He took the book back to school with him to work through again by himself. This was really the first attempt at reading he made although he had done little bits on his own before. Since then he has been prepared to read books about technical matters which interest him. (But still at nineteen years cannot read aloud from the newspaper with any confidence.)

"He retained his conviction that he would not be able to do maths until he had to accept the necessity for learning the subject in connection with his interest in electronics. He got through his 'O' level in maths and then, much to my surprise, opted to study both pure and applied maths for 'A' levels. He now says that he finds the subject enjoyable.

"I am convinced that, if we had not acted when we did to take him out of the school situation he might well have been in a mental hospital by now. He was getting more and more depressed, and was withdrawing from contact with the outside world into a world of his own. I think that if the outside pressures had continued for much longer he might have eventually withdrawn altogether.

"[in 1969 he] passed 'O' level technical drawing but did a complete mirror image of one of the drawings asked for—a much more difficult task than the question required... [in 1970 he] failed 'O' level in English Language, re-sat, and failed again ... is about to sit 'O' level advanced maths, and to re-sit English."

In addition to confirming that Robert was dyslexic, I wrote a certificate which I hoped would be passed on to the appropriate examination boards. After the initial preamble I said: "He is likely to be slow, because of his disability, at reading examination questions and slow at checking calculations. He is 'at risk' in that he may go 'off the rails' with miscopying or misunderstanding unless he spends a disproportionate amount of time checking. The final result may therefore not be a reflection of his true ability.

"Could I recommend, therefore, (*a*) that he be given extra time, and (*b*) that examiners be alerted to the possibility of anomalous results, and that his scripts be considered in this light."

Robert's first attempt at 'A' level resulted in passes at the lowest grade in both Pure and Applied Mathematics and a fail in Physics. In a letter which he wrote to me at the time he said that his tutor had noticed that in examinations he always chose the *shortest* questions, i.e. those which required less reading, rather than the *easiest* ones.

I still felt that Robert should be encouraged to go to university. When I wrote back, I said: "It is annoying about the low grades, as obviously your *ability* is much more. But our experience here is that many people with dyslexia have persevered and passed exams even after quite a number of 'fails' or low-grade passes."

When I was approached by the University to which

Robert had applied I wrote: "I hope —— University will be able to accept him. I regard him as a very deserving case. Like many sufferers from dyslexia he has fought a real battle against the educational system, and this has called for both ability and determination.

"My suggestion would be that the Department concerned give him a thorough interview. He himself will be able to describe accurately his past difficulties and any residual effects which still exist. His spelling is still rather poor and he may take marginally longer than others in the actual mechanics of reading, though his quick intellect is an important compensation here. He is 'at risk' in that it may take him longer to check that he has copied things correctly; if he rushes he might get circuit-diagrams the wrong way round, for instance. At an earlier stage simple computation was not easy for him ... If the University is flexible in its examination system, he could be helped enormously e.g. by being given more time or in other ways. In a rigid conventional exam, where one is timed and has to check calculations, he is bound to be handicapped, and I don't doubt this explains his low 'A' level grades, which probably represent the combined effect of high ability with slowness at reading, slowness at calculation, and slowness at getting things down. Presumably at university level one is glad to have mathematicians and is less concerned as to whether they are quick at calculation!

"In view of his ability I don't myself feel a university would be running any serious risk by accepting him, but I recommend a thorough interview, so that those who will be teaching him can be clear where his difficulties used to lie and will not be surprised if residual difficulties still show themselves."

Happily, Robert was accepted by the University in question, and when he repeated his 'A' level examinations he obtained grades B, D, and D instead of the E, E, and Fail of his previous attempt.

There are a number of comments which I should like to make on this case. First, the degree of understanding which Robert's mother showed was quite unusual. I have met many families where something was already known about dyslexia, in particular an appreciation that "something odd" is happening and that the child is not just being obstinate and difficult for no reason. In these cases one can "fit the pieces together" for the parents, so that they can appreciate, for example, that problems over left and right and problems of memorizing arithmetical tables are all part of the dyslexia. In the case of Robert's mother, however, there was very little that I could tell her which she did not know already; and it is perhaps ironic that she clearly knew more about dyslexia than the "experts" at the child guidance clinic who were supposed to be advising her.

I have sometimes heard the sneer that "dyslexia" is a label used by middle-class parents to obtain preferential treatment for less able children. Yet many parents have said to me, as Robert's mother did, "We did not want to worry if his slow progress was due to low intelligence;" and I have met some dyslexic children whose parents did not know about dyslexia at all—and who could scarcely, therefore, be using the word for selfish or disreputable purposes! There have, of course, been parents who have been upset and distressed at their child's sufferings and as a result have had plenty to say; but it seems to me that if their child is dyslexic they have every right to take the matter seriously. To dismiss such people as over-fussy seems to me quite criminal.

Where a dyslexic child has been "put off" reading and spelling, one helpful procedure is to encourage him with things that he can do well. Sometimes this is art, while in Robert's case it was pottery and playing the drum and the guitar. It is also very important to remember that those who are weak at calculation and remembering tables can none the less be very competent mathematicians.

Robert's story has a reasonably happy ending. One cannot but think, however, that a large amount of suffering could have been avoided had his teachers known something about dyslexia when he first went to school. In the next chapter I shall try to make some general statements as to how a dyslexic child, such as Robert, John, Henry or Laura, can be picked out.

Recognizing Dyslexia

TO introduce the subject of recognizing, or "diagnosing," dyslexia it will be helpful, I think, to start by reconsidering some of the difficulties experienced by Henry, John, Laura and Robert.

None of them was stupid, yet in each case there were mistakes which were altogether surprising in view of their general intellectual ability. In all four cases there had been difficulties with reading and spelling which to varying extents had been overcome. All four still had problems, though not identical ones, over left and right, and all four were weak at various kinds of arithmetical computation. Henry, John and Laura all had difficulty in saying digits in reverse order (a test not given to Robert); Robert continually needed to have things repeated and is reported to have produced a complete mirror-image in a technical drawing test; John was said to have a very insecure sense of time, and so on.

In view of all this, it is perhaps helpful to regard dyslexia as a *family* of difficulties. Not every dyslexic sign is present in every case and similar mistakes may occasionally be made by those who are not dyslexic, but a person can be regarded as "dyslexic" if a sufficient number of these signs occur together.

As already pointed out (p. 15), a dyslexic child can learn to compensate for some of his difficulties. This necessarily makes the problem of diagnosis more complicated. A particular child may succeed in a task where other dyslexic children have failed simply because he has been clever enough to devise a compensatory strategy. Thus John surprised me by his ability to repeat such polysyllabic words as "preliminary" and "statistical," a task which almost all of those with dyslexia find difficult; but from his remarks it seemed likely that by looking at the syllables of Spanish words in detail he had somehow learned to study the parts of longer words in isolation. One cannot therefore infer that he had never had any potential limitation over repeating such words; it is possible that he had had this limitation and had learned to overcome it. What one meets on any particular occasion with a dyslexic child may sometimes be a sort of composite: he may have had all kinds of potential limitations, and one may be testing him at a stage when he has learned to overcome some of them and not others. To make things even more complicated, a non-dyslexic child may fail the same test item not because of any specific handicap but simply because it is too difficult for him.

By derivation "dyslexia" means "difficulty with language;" "*dys*" is the Greek root meaning "difficulty with" and "*lexis*," connected with the root "*logos*," means something like "language," "speech," or "diction." Confusion has arisen, however, because people have associated it with the Latin word "*lego*," meaning "read," and have therefore assumed that "dyslexia" means "difficulty with reading."

Derivations are not necessarily important, but this particular confusion has been unfortunate, since it has led people to suppose that if a child can read fairly well then he cannot be dyslexic. In many dyslexic children correct reading is in fact a relatively minor problem (though quite a number are slow at reading). More often it is spelling which presents special difficulty, at least in the early stages; and the emphasis on poor reading diverts attention both from spelling difficulties and from the difficulties over arithmetic, space and time which have been mentioned above. Indeed, the substitution of "reading difficulty" for "dyslexia" results in misclassification, since there are many people who are poor readers without being dyslexic and many people who are dyslexic and yet are adequate readers.

There is no special mystique in picking out a dyslexic child. Although examining boards and other authorities are no doubt correct in insisting that an actual certificate of dyslexia should be signed by a suitably trained doctor or educational psychologist, the recognition itself seems to me to be well within the competence of the average parent or teacher, provided only that he or she knows what to look for. I shall therefore set out the relevant diagnostic signs in the hope that they will not only be of use to doctors and educational psychologists in their professional work but also be of interest to the layman who wishes to know more about how a diagnosis of dyslexia is made.

In brief, a person is dyslexic provided (*a*) that there is a discrepancy between his intellectual level and his performance at reading or spelling and (*b*) that this discrepancy is accompanied by some of the supporting "signs" which have been mentioned.

A word of warning is necessary at this point, however. One cannot expect a dyslexic child to make the same mistake on all occasions. For example, if you have been told that a child sometimes writes b for d in spelling or sometimes misreads t as d, you cannot be sure that he will make this kind of mistake when next tested. It seems more correct to say that the dyslexic child is vulnerable and therefore *liable* to make this kind of mistake even if he does not *always* do so. The same is true of other kinds of dyslexic mistakes. If he never makes any such mistakes he is not dyslexic; it is quite common, however, for a dyslexic child to misread or misspell a word on one occasion and not on another, or fail at a "digits-reversed" test on, say, his first and third attempts but not on his second attempt. It is important, therefore, to look out for *inconsistencies* of performance, and not always be content with results when a task is given on one occasion only.

A necessary procedure at the start is to obtain an estimate of the child's ability at reading and spelling. Various tests can be used for this purpose. In the case of reading there are, for example, the tests by Schonell, Daniels and Diack, and Neale, while Schonell and also Daniels and Diack have prepared tests of spelling. Details of all these tests are given in Appendix I, p. 125–6. If no such tests are available you may be able to obtain limited information by asking the child to read from a book that is to hand or to spell some words of your own choosing; but, unless his performance is a long way outside normal limits it is hard by this means to be sure

51

if there is any appreciable backwardness. The actual score on a standardized test will be a more accurate guide, though in addition to counting the number of right and wrong answers it is helpful to observe in detail the kinds of mistake which he makes, the time which he takes, his false starts and corrections, his hesitations, the amount of confidence which he shows, and so on.

His "reading age" and "spelling age," however, will be of help only if you know his actual age and something about his intelligence level. This is, in fact, an example of a general point which holds good for the diagnosis as a whole: *the meaning of a particular sign will depend on the context in which it occurs.* Thus, if you find—or are told—that he spelled 45 words correctly on the Schonell test and thus has a spelling age of 9.5, this means something different according to whether he is, for example, an average 7-year old, a dull 11-year old, or a bright 12-year old. If he is only 7 and can already spell to this level, it would be fairly safe to exclude dyslexia then and there; if he is a dull 11-year old, it is possible that you may find some dyslexic signs if you look for them; if he is a bright 12-year-old, then you can say at once that there is a discrepancy betweeen intellectual level and performance at spelling, and this would lead you positively to *expect* further dyslexic signs. Even then, of course, it is important to be flexible and not to let your expectations affect the objectivity of your observations. If you conclude that the child is dyslexic, you are saying, in effect, that he has certain constitutional limitations; and if this is true, these limitations will show themselves in other ways, such as difficulty over putting things in sequence, difficulty in repeating digits reversed, etc. If no such "supporting signs" occur, you will clearly need to think again.

Knowing something about the child's intelligence level is essential for accurate diagnosis. The whole question of intelligence and intelligence testing, however, is a controversial one. My personal view is that the notion of an "I.Q." ("intelligence quotient") has been over-rated and that placing people on a uni-dimensional scale in respect of the relative "amount" that they possess of whatever-it-is is fundamentally misguided. Intelligence tests comprise a variety of different tasks, and adding up a person's successes in them is quite unlike measuring his height or taking his temperature. I myself, therefore, am opposed to the use of the I.Q. if it is thought of as a "measure" of the amount of intellectual ability which a person possesses. It may be interesting to see which particular reasoning tasks he finds easy or difficult and I do not dispute the need to use intelligence tests for some purposes. What I do object to is the assumption that one is thereby "measuring" some uni-dimensional quality. I readily allow, however, that there are those who would wish to read more into the notion of an I.Q. than I do.

As far as a diagnosis of dyslexia is concerned, the main use of the results of an intelligence test is as a means of excluding dullness as the main cause of the child's educational difficulties. Clearly, a dull child may not be able to repeat long words correctly and may have difficulty in saying three or four digits backwards; and such failures are therefore positive signs of dyslexia only if dullness has been excluded. I shall say more later about dull children who make dyslexic-type mistakes (see pp 75 seq.), but at this point all that is needed is to stress that their requirements are different from those of the typical dyslexic child whose intellectual level and spelling performance are discrepant.

If you know enough about what to expect from a typical child of a given age, then clearly you can form *some* estimate of his ability simply from listening to him talk. Thus if a 10-year old tells you about transistors or a 12-year old about the plot of King Lear, there would be a strong presumption from this evidence alone that neither is dull; but, as in the case of reading and spelling, standardized tests give you results upon which you can act with greater confidence. I am not saying that the I.Q. figure is a genuine measure of something whereas the result of listening to the child or giving him an improvised test is not; but the advantage of using tests from which I.Q. figures are derived is that these tests have been standardized.

Quite apart from general problems about the significance of I.Q. figures, there are special problems about ascribing such figures to those with dyslexia. In general, "group" tests of intelligence, that is pencil and paper tests administered to a group of children at a time, are unsatisfactory. Even in so-called "non-verbal" tests the child may still sometimes be required to read the instructions, while in "verbal" tests, which necessarily call for the reading of written material, a dyslexic child may misread what is there or, if he tries to avoid this by being extra careful, may go very slowly; and in a timed test, he will then end up with a score that does not genuinely reflect his ability. In any case there is not the chance in a group test to watch the child in detail and find out, for instance, which answers are difficult for him, why they are difficult, how he reacts to success and failure, and so on. When told that the child's I.Q. figure is so-and-so, you would be wise to ask what particular test was used, and if the figure is based on the result of a group test it is particularly advisable to treat it with caution.

The two most important intelligence tests which are given to children individually are the Wechsler Intelligence Scale for Children (usually abbreviated to W.I.S.C.) and the Stanford Binet (known also as the Terman-Merrill or as the Terman for short*). Details of these tests are given in Appendix I, p. 125. But even if one of these two tests has been used, the difficulties in assessing the intelligence of a dyslexic child are not over. When the tests were published the needs of those with dyslexia do not appear to have been considered. Experience now suggests that there are some items which dyslexic children can do perfectly well and others which they regularly find difficult.

Let us take the W.I.S.C. first. This test is divided into two halves, known respectively as the "verbal" and "performance" halves. The verbal half contains a section termed "Information," which includes such questions as "Who discovered America?," a section called "Comprehension," which includes such questions as, "What should you do if you see a train approaching a broken railway

---

* Professors Terman and Merrill, of Stanford University, were responsible for adapting and modifying a set of tests originally devised by the French psychologist, Alfred Binet.

line?," a test involving arithmetical calculations, a vocabulary test, a test in which the child has to say how two thing are alike, for example "cat" and "mouse," and a memory test in which the child has to repeat a string of digits after they have been spoken by the tester, followed by a second section in which the digits have to be repeated in reverse order. The "performance" half of the W.I.S.C. contains a section called "Picture Completion," in which the child is given a picture incomplete in some way and has to say what is missing, a section called "Picture Arrangement," when cards have to be arranged in such a way that they tell a coherent story, a section called "Block Design," in which the child uses blocks to copy the pattern presented on a card, a section called "Object Assembly," in which the child has to make a representation of a horse, a motor-car, etc. from component parts, and a section called "Coding" in which the child has to attach the appropriate symbol, for example a dot or a line, to particular digits in accordance with rules given to him.

On the basis of research by Naidoo (1972, p. 56; see Further Reading, p. 136, no. 13) there are grounds for saying that dyslexic children find some of these sub-tests harder than others. I shall not attempt a detailed account of Mrs. Naidoo's procedure; but one of the things which she did in her research was compare the performance of two groups of dyslexic children (they were classed as "dyslexic" by carefully specified criteria) with the performance of two "control" groups—children matched for age and social background with the dyslexic groups but not retarded in reading or spelling. The main findings can be roughly summarized as follows: the dyslexic children scored lower than the control children on the information and vocabulary sub-tests and appreciably lower on the arithmetic, digit span and coding sub-tests. In contrast there were fewer differences—and in some cases virtually none at all—on the comprehension, similarities, picture completion, picture arrangement and block design sub-tests.

From what we know of dyslexia most of these results are not surprising. As already stated in Chapter 1, tests involving memory for digits, as well as some arithmetical calculations, are regularly found to present difficulty to dyslexic children. Also, in view of what many of them miss through lack of reading, it is not at all unexpected that they should score lower than the controls on the information sub-test. In contrast there is nothing in most of the items in the comprehension and picture completion sub-tests which would be specially likely to cause difficulty. In the case of the vocabulary sub-test it seems possible that two separate factors are at work: a dyslexic child's vocabulary may be wide because he is alert and has picked up the use of fairly sophisticated words in the home, yet it may be narrow because he has done far less reading than a non-dyslexic child of the same age. His score may therefore be a sort of composite, being determined in part by the kind of spoken vocabulary to which he has been exposed.

I know of no comparable evidence about the performance of dyslexic children on the Terman test, but I have found in my own experience that similar considerations apply. Thus most of them are likely to be successful with problems involving similarities and moderately successful on "vocabulary"; but many are likely to have difficulty with tests involving arithmetical calculation, and the majority can be expected to have difficulty over saying digits in reverse.

The conclusion seems inevitable: one cannot simply take I.Q. figures at their face-value. Certain types of failure, e.g. over "digits reversed," can be regarded as positive indicators of dyslexia, whereas certain types of success, for instance in items which involve abstract reasoning, show what the child can do in areas not affected by his dyslexia. To add these two together to make a composite I.Q. figure scarcely seems helpful. Indeed it would be true to say that one can actually *make* the I.Q. figure high or low according to the tests used.

There is a further complication. If one presents an I.Q. figure, this implies that one knows what it means or what can be done with it. Now in the normal way the I.Q. figure is used as a prediction of likely scholastic attainment, and those who score highly are normally encouraged to do courses with an academic bias. If, therefore, one's purpose in presenting the I.Q. figure of a dyslexic child is to make predictions about future academic success, it immediately becomes plain that one is on unsafe ground. Indeed, as we shall see more fully in Chapter 8, it is not at all easy to predict what a dyslexic child will achieve academically; much depends on the extent to which he has the opportunity to learn ways of compensating for his disability.

I am not, of course, saying that the Wechsler and Terman tests should never be used with dyslexic children.

What I am attacking is the uncritical use of I.Q. figures. It is, of course, perfectly reasonable to use the test results as evidence for excluding general dullness. If an 11-year old passes several items at the "average adult" level on the Terman test dullness one can rule out with complete confidence. Similarly, if he performs at a level which is average for his age on the Wechsler similarities or picture completion tests, one can again exclude dullness. Indeed, evidence of any kind which indicates that he is capable of difficult reasoning tasks is highly relevant and it is this kind of evidence which one can hope to obtain from the use of traditional intelligence tests.

This, then, is the first stage in the diagnosis: it is necessary to find out whether there is a discrepancy between the child's intellectual level and his performance at spelling. If there is not, then one may conclude that he is not a serious or typical case of dyslexia.

In most cases reading as well as spelling will usually be weaker than would be expected from the child's intellectal level, but it is a mistake to rely too heavily on the child's reading age as a diagnostic sign, since some dyslexic children—particularly those lucky enough to have received skilled and intensive teaching—can read fairly well; in these cases the dyslexia may be masked by a good performance at reading. I have also met really bright children whose reading age is on a level with their actual age or even above it but who none the less are dyslexic. One is sure that they are dyslexic from the presence of many other dyslexic signs, and they are, of course, still "discrepant" in the sense that their performance at reading, though not behind what is average for their age, is still behind what would be expected from their intelligence level. Such children are sometimes regarded as being average in ability by their teachers when in fact their average performance is a composite of extreme brightness coupled with dyslexia. Any educational survey which relies solely on scores on a reading test is likely to miss a number of children who are in fact dyslexic (cf. pp. 97 seq.).

Another thing to watch for is so-called "bizarre" spelling. Plenty of examples appear in Chapter 1, for example Henry's "elestricaty" for "electricity" and John's "pniced" for "panicked" and "marie on Twanet" for "Marie Antoinette." Sometimes parts of the word are left out; sometimes letters are put in the wrong order; sometimes there is intelligent but quite mistaken phonetic spelling, and sometimes several of these things happen in combination—in which case the effect is even more weird. This "bizarre" spelling is easier to recognize than to describe, and from an examination of the child's school books—including those of an earlier stage if they are still available—the tester will normally have little difficulty in discovering if it is present.

The next stage in the diagnosis is to see if some of the accompanying dyslexic signs are present.

The first of these which I should like to mention is confusion between b and d. Once again one needs to bear in mind the age and intelligence of the child. Before the age of about $7\frac{1}{2}$ such confusions can be regarded as possible warning signs, but cannot be regarded as decisive evidence of dyslexia. After the age of 8, however, few non-dyslexic children of average ability display these confusions; and it follows that if you are dealing with a bright 8- or 9-year old who has other dyslexic signs, the presence of b-d confusion will be further confirmation that he is dyslexic. In the case of other children, that is those of 12 and upwards, it is possible that they themselves will not remember that they ever confused b and d, though I have sometimes discovered afterwards from talking to their parents that in fact they did so at an earlier stage.

It is also important to check whether b-d confusion occurs in both reading and writing or whether it occurs in writing only. (I do not know of any cases where it has occurred in reading only, but this is not to say that no such cases exist.) If one is inspecting school books for bizarre spelling it is helpful to look out for b-d confusion at the same time.

The next stage in the diagnosis is to see if the child has a clear conception of left and right. It may be helpful, even in the case of older children and adults, to start with a simple request such as "Show me your right hand." Even here one occasionally finds surprising results—a significant pause or the invoking of a special mnemonic. In the case of more articulate children one may sometimes be told, "I used to get very muddled" or even "I've learned now—the *right* hand is the one I *write* with," or "It's the hand with the scar [or ring] on," or "I know my watch is on my left hand, so my right must be the other one." A more difficult task is involved if, sitting opposite the child, you say, "Which is my right hand?" or "Point to my left ear with your right hand." In recent months, however, I have become somewhat less confident about the value of such tests for picking out dyslexic children, since it is possible that the task is difficult for some non-dyslexic children too. If, therefore, there were few other positive signs in the rest of the assessment one would be wrong, I am sure, to attach too much import-ance to a failure on such tests. If, however, it is accom-panied by other signs of dyslexia, one may reasonably regard such failure as additional evidence that the child is dyslexic.

Some years ago, after giving the Schonell reading test to a number of older dyslexic children, I happened to notice that most of them were stumbling over the word "preliminary." I have since noticed that various other longer words seem to cause difficulty, for example "statis-tical," "philosophical" and "anemone," (often repeated as "an enemy"). Some rough surveys have indicated that quite a large number of 9-year olds may have difficulty in correctly repeating words of this complexity, but in a bright child of 10 or more it seems perfectly safe to regard such failure as a positive sign of dyslexia. This is confirmed by a study of the attempts which dyslexic children make at spelling "preliminary": syllables are omitted and letters are confused in a most curious way. The following are examples from our Bangor records: "plemerrley," "premerriley," "pellimery," "preliary," "plerminary," "plemerly" and "pliminary."

When dyslexic children are asked to say these longer words there is often the same sequence of behaviour: they make an attempt which is somewhere near correct, and if you then ask them to repeat the word they say part of it and then hesitate and become confused. At this point they may smile in a sheepish way, sometimes with an indication of exasperation at their failure. It is as though both of you were acknowledging the incongruity—and perhaps even the humour—of this kind of failure.

It has been mentioned already that those with dyslexia seem to have special difficulty in saying digits in reverse order. To check on this I have found it helpful to adapt the procedure used in the Wechsler test: I tell the child that I will be saying some numbers and that he is to say them backwards, and he is then given an example for practice, such as, "If I were to say 4-2-7, what would you say?" If he replies "7-2-4" then he has grasped what is required. The digits should be presented at the rate of about one per second. If the child has difficulty outside normal limits, this again is a positive indication of dyslexia. Experience is perhaps the main guide as to what are "normal limits," but as a rough indication it is worth noting that the Terman test (which has been given to many thousands of children) puts "four digits reversed" at age 9, "five digits reversed" at age 12, and "six digits reversed" at the first grade of "superior adult." As with many tests for dyslexia, however, interest lies less in correctness as such than in the way in which the child sets to work. I have met very few dyslexic children who have failed at three digits reversed on every trial, but I have met plenty who have failed at, say, two attempts out of three. Throughout the diagnosis one is trying to find whether the child is *vulnerable* at a particular task, not whether he can occasionally produce the right answer.

I have also found it useful to ask the child to say the months of the year. Some dyslexic children can do this task successfully, but quite a number either omit months

63

or put them in the wrong order. Older children and adults can be asked to say the months of the year backwards, and it will soon be apparent if the person has any unusual difficulty. Once again correctness is not the main thing to watch for; a very bright dyslexic child may be able to bring in all sorts of compensatory devices as a result of which the correct answer emerges, but if for instance, before answering he said them forwards under his breath, one would certainly be entitled to say that the condition of "unusual difficulty" was satisfied.

A few dyslexic children have difficulty with numbers. They cannot, for instance, do subtraction unless they first represent the numbers in concrete form—by counting on their fingers, for instance, or by using marks on paper or beads or blocks. This, however, is not typical of the majority.

What is far more common is difficulty in remembering and reciting arithmetical tables. This is one of the areas in which dyslexic children have continually been dubbed "lazy," but the difficulty is so widespread that it cannot be accidental. Most of them can remember the obvious products, such as 2×3, and, where there is a clear rule, as in the case of the ten-times and eleven-times tables, they are able to apply it. What is difficult for them is to answer on the spot such questions as "What is 6×7?" or "What is 8×7?" (compare the report of the conversation with John, p. 31). In addition, if asked to recite tables in the traditional way, for example "One six is six, two sixes are twelve," they are liable to lose their place, perhaps by passing from five sixes to seven sixes, or to hesitate and say "Where have I got to?" This "where-have-I-got-to?" response occurs fairly regularly even with older dyslexic children.

Some dyslexic children are reported as being unusually clumsy and some are said to have been late at walking and/or talking. Although these signs do not occur in every case, they are sufficiently frequent to be regarded as confirmatory evidence that the child is dyslexic, provided some of the main dyslexic signs are also present.

The following, then, are some of the main signs of dyslexia to look out for:
(i) discrepancy between intellectual level and performance at spelling, (ii) bizarre spelling, (iii) confusion of b and d in either reading or writing, or in both, (iv) difficulty over distinguishing left and right, (v) difficulty in repeating polysyllabic words, such as "preliminary," "philosophical," "statistical," and "anemone," (vi) difficulty in repeating digits in reverse order (and other defects of short term memory), (vii) difficulty in repeating months of the year, especially in reverse order, (viii) inability to do subtractions except with "concrete" aids, (ix) difficulty in memorizing arithmetical tables, (x) "losing the place" when reciting tables, (xi) a history of clumsiness, late walking, or late talking.

Not all these signs will be present in any one child, but if the original discrepancy between intellectual level and performance at spelling is accompanied by two or three others it is safe to say that the child is dyslexic; and this is, in effect, to say that his educational difficulties have a constitutional basis.

If possible, it is also helpful to try to discover if any

65

other members of the family have had similar difficulties. There are plenty of occasions when the result may be negative, but if it is positive one's confidence that this particular child is dyslexic is very much increased. The question of the incidence of dyslexia in families will be discussed further in Chapter 4.

3

Doubtful Cases

THERE are plenty of cases where it is possible to say without hesitation that a child is dyslexic. Occasionally, however, I have been in the situation where I was unsure whether the child was genuinely dyslexic or not.

One can, of course, be doubtful about how to designate a child for a variety of reasons. For instance, if one needs data for research purposes an extra degree of caution is desirable simply as a safety measure; to include "doubtful" cases in one's statistical tables is to run the risk of drawing faulty conclusions. There may be other situations, however, where the reason for doubt is not academic caution but a genuine uncertainty as to how a particular child can best be helped. In the case of a dyslexic child the basic requirement is specialist individual teaching, and while one can envisage few occasions where such a programme would do positive harm if the child turned out not to be dyslexic, there might be situations where it was irrelevant and therefore time-wasting. In particular, if resources are limited, one wants to be sure that specialist skills are going to those who need them most.

The semantic problems in this area are awkward. One is sometimes tempted to say, "Provided people agree that the child needs help then the name given to his difficulties does not matter." This, however, is unsatisfactory. Words serve to classify and while it is unimportant which of two words is used if they are synonymous and therefore carry the same implications, there may be situations where the wrong use of a word results in a wrong classification, and here the consequences can be extremely serious. For example, the terms "dyslexia," "specific language disability," and "word-blindness" are all approximately synonymous, and which expression we use is relatively unimportant. "Dyslexia" and "reading difficulty," however, are not synonymous: not all those who have difficulty in reading are dyslexic; some of those who are dyslexic can read quite well (even if reading did not come easily in the first place) and all have difficulties other than reading. To classify "poor readers" together as a single group is to ignore these important differences.

Even if this point is recognized, however, the semantic problems are not over: doubts about whether a particular person is dyslexic are not always due to factual uncertainty. To quote a phrase used by the philosopher, Wittgenstein, in a different context: "We do not know the boundaries because none have been drawn." If we apply Wittgenstein's dictum to the notion of "dyslexia" it becomes plain that nobody has ever laid down what precisely is to *count as* being dyslexic. If therefore, we choose to stipulate what are to be the correct criteria we need to be clear as to the purpose of the classification which is being made. One may sometimes be quite sure of the relevant facts while still being unsure how best to describe them. Perhaps we should speak here of a "semantic" uncertainty, as opposed to a "factual" uncertainty. It is as though someone had a clear view of a flower in ordinary daylight but was still unsure whether its colour—which he could clearly see—was to count as, say, yellow or green.

There are four main types of situation where I have felt doubt as to whether or not someone should be called "dyslexic." (1) The first is the situation where such a person is virtually a non-reader and non-speller and where there is therefore no possibility of studying the kinds of mistakes which he makes. (2) The second is the situation where results on reading and spelling tests are somewhat below average, but where the other signs, such as difficulty over distinguishing left and right, difficulty in saying tables, and so on, are so mild as hardly to be outside normal limits. (3) The third is the situation where dyslexic-type mistakes such as b-d confusion are fairly frequent, but where there is no serious discrepancy between intellectual level and performance at reading and spelling. (4) The fourth is the situation where a child has some kind of similar learning "block," for example in arithmetic, but has relatively less trouble with reading or spelling.

In the first two situations one simply needs more facts (which may or may not become available), while in the third and fourth one is involved in what is partly an issue of semantics, since in effect one has first to settle the general question of *when to call* a person "dyslexic." These semantic issues, however, are often extremely important, since if we decide to talk in a certain way we are thereby opting for a particular classification and hence for a particular policy. Each of these four situations will be considered in turn.

(1) A few years ago a man in his forties came to see me. He could write only a few letters and could not read any words apart from "a," "the," and a few others. An intelligence test showed him to be of average ability and there seemed to be no reason in his previous history (such as lack of opportunity or physical defect) why he had not learned to read and spell. He said that at school he had sat at the back of the class and kept clear of serious trouble. At the present time he was employed as a painter. To avoid having to read or write in public he had sometimes invented "lost glasses" or a "broken wrist," and though he could not write "wet paint" he had been able to manage "WET." From what he told me it was impossible to say whether or not he was dyslexic. Indeed, if in general one knows only that a person cannot read or spell and very little else, there are insufficient grounds for either diagnosing or excluding dyslexia. When he came for special teaching, however, and started to write words such as "big," "bad," and "dog," I found that he was regularly confusing b and d. This immediately created a strong presumption that he was dyslexic, or in other words that his difficulties were due to a constitutional limitation (with presumably a physiological basis). This presumption will turn into a certainty if further dyslexic-type mistakes occur. No issue of semantics is involved here; at present I am unsure simply because I have insufficient evidence. Here is another case where again, the evidence is incomplete.

Recently, a mother asked me to see her daughter, Elspeth, aged 6 years 2 months. I explained that I would be unable to say at such a young age whether or not Elspeth was dyslexic; but her mother, who was familiar with the relevant literature, thought that a definite disability was present and asked me to do what I could.

When given the Terman intelligence test Elspeth passed three items at the 8-year level, and in general her performance was above average for a 6-year old. Her reading age came out as 6.4 and her spelling age as 6.2. At first glance, therefore, one might suppose that, since she was not behind her age-level at reading and spelling, there was no special cause for concern. Moreover the fact that she failed to point to my left and right sides as I sat opposite her and failed to repeat the words "preliminary" and "statistical" was not evidence for dyslexia since any 6-year old would find such tasks difficult.

When I looked in detail, however, at what she could and could not do, I realized that her mother's fears were very far from being groundless. (In general, my experience is that when observant parents feel that there is something wrong or incongruous about a child's performance at reading and spelling they are more than likely to be right; and if one fails to take such feelings seriously one is not only being uncharitable but also running considerable risk of being mistaken.) Elspeth had in fact correctly spelled the straightforward words from the Schonell test, "can," "hit," "lid," and so on, but one cannot therefore exclude the possibility of dyslexia, since these words are phonetically regular and with phonetically irregular words it is possible that she will have far more difficulty. Similarly, just because she can read fourteen of the words in the Schonell word-recognition test it certainly does not follow that reading in general will be no problem. She in fact wrote "gg" for "egg" and "ysy" for "yes," which are unusual mistakes, to say the least. Also there seemed to be some evidence of a difficulty over sequencing: when asked to say the months of the year she showed considerable hesitation and finally said "December, November, April, July;" and when asked to say the seasons of the year she said "Winter, autumn, spring, autumn, winter." Although she repeated the days of the week correctly forwards, when asked to say them backwards she said "Saturday, Sunday, Friday," then, with long pauses, "Thursday, Wednesday," and with even longer pauses "Tuesday, Monday." While one cannot say for certain that such responses are outside normal limits for a bright 6-year old, the general "feel" of the situation suggests that they are. Even where norms are available, as in the case of the digits reversed test, the conclusion is not clear-cut. In this test Elspeth was successful on one out of three trials, which means, according to the Terman norms, that she just passes at the vii-year level. In other words, we have a minimal pass at year vii from a girl who passed several other items at year viii with ease. I readily allow that the evidence for her being dyslexic was inconclusive, but it was certainly not negligible. In my report, therefore, I suggested that her teachers should be on the look out for an *incongruous* performance and that at the very least she should be regarded as being "at risk."

This, then, is another case where there was insufficient information. At the time of writing I do not know whether in the next few years Elspeth is going to display the typical dyslexic difficulties. It is, of course, possible that if she is re-tested at, say, age nine, the teaching which she has received in the meantime will cause a few of her difficulties to be masked; but if she is genuinely dyslexic this means by definition that at least some of the signs described in Chapter 2 will be found. If none are present, it follows that one was wrong to regard her as being at risk. If, however, there are still incongruities, at least in the things which she has not practised, then even if she has learned to read adequately it does not follow that she is not dyslexic, only that by hard effort she has in part learned to compensate for her disability. In Elspeth's case I am not sure if she is dyslexic because I do not know what difficulties she will be having in two or three years' time.

(2) One may also feel doubt in the situation where some of the typically dyslexic signs are present, for example difficulty in repeating polysyllabic words or in remembering arithmetical tables, but where one is unsure if this weakness is outside normal limits.

James was referred to me at the age of 8¾. He came out as average on the Wechsler intelligence test; his "reading age" on the Schonell word-recognition test was 7¾ and his "spelling age" was three months lower. (These figures represent 89% and 86%, respectively, of his actual age.) He made two mistakes in six trials when asked to point to the left or right sides of my body as I sat opposite him; he failed to repeat a number of polysyllabic words, such as "preliminary" and "statistical"; he made one mistake in a subtraction test; he showed slight signs of "losing his place" in reciting his four-times and five-times tables and I found "on" written as "no" in one of his school books.

His difficulty over left and right and his difficulty over the polysyllabic words were neither of them, in my judgment, outside normal limits, and the single mistake in the subtraction test is quite inconclusive. The confusion of "on" and "no" is unusual in an 8-year old of average ability, and the difficulty with tables surprised me. But, that apart, there seemed very little on which to base a diagnosis of dyslexia, particularly since his performance in the reading and spelling tests was not all that far behind the average for his age. When I looked in detail at the sub-test scores on the Wechsler test, I found that the typical dyslexic patterning (cf. p. 57) was largely absent: although weak on the coding test, like many dyslexic children, he had a high score on digit span (which is extremely unusual in a dyslexic child) and low scores on comprehension and similarities (where almost all dyslexic children score relatively highly).

I think one must conclude that James is not a typical case of dyslexia one could perhaps say that he showed a few dyslexic signs. In fact it was possible to arrange some special reading and spelling lessons for him in which he was taught words containing the letters "oo," "oi," "igh," (for example "soon," "boil," "might") and other words which "go the same way." His teacher indicated that he had less of a struggle than most of the typically dyslexic children whom she had taught.

I have met very few "marginal" cases of this kind and I am not sure whether there is a reasonably clear "cut-off point" between those who are dyslexic and those who are not, or whether there are all degrees of handicap from "zero" to "very severe." I think it possible that some of those who have an inherited constitutional weakness (and hence are, if you like, "potentially" dyslexic) have learned to compensate so effectively that almost no signs remain. Such compensation, if it has occurred, would admittedly be difficult to distinguish from normal growth, but it seems to me not impossible that some children who appear as marginal cases are in fact children who were constitutionally at risk but have learned to compensate. This, however, is somewhat speculative.

The fact that there is uncertainty over marginal cases does not, of course, mean that a dyslexic child and a non-dyslexic child are no different!

(3) A further set of problems is raised by the fact that many children at special schools or in special remedial classes (so-called "slow learning" children) sometimes show the same difficulties as the dyslexic child. In particular, confusions between b and d are common among such children, and it is likely that many would show the same difficulties as dyslexic children over reciting tables, saying months of the year, and similar tests. If these difficulties are the defining characteristic of dyslexia, must one not conclude that large numbers of slow-learning children are dyslexic?

An important criterion commonly used in deciding

whether or not a child is dyslexic is that of "discrepancy." One looks, in other words, to see if there is something *discrepant* about the child's performance, and in particular to see whether there is a difference between intellectual level on the one hand and performance at reading and spelling on the other.

In the case of children in special schools it is particularly important to check in the first place whether this "discrepancy criterion" is or is not satisfied. The fact that a child does poorly in certain tests involving the use of language does not entitle one to conclude, *ipso facto*, that he "has a low I.Q." In such cases some of the items from the performance half of the Wechsler test should certainly be given, for example the picture completion and block design tests. If an apparently slow child is somewhere near average on these tests and yet is considerably behind the standard for his age-level at reading or spelling, then the discrepancy criterion is satisfied, and, if other supporting signs are present, he would count as a genuine case of dyslexia.

There may, however, be other situations where the child's mistakes are "dyslexic" in character (b-d confusion, etc.) but where there is no serious discrepancy. Here, I think, there are advantages in making the "discrepancy criterion" a necessary condition for a diagnosis of dyslexia. Admittedly, for all we know, it may be that someone who confuses b and d is similar, physiologically, to someone else who confuses b and d. At present, however, we do not know enough about physiology for this point to be of practical relevance. What is important, it seems to me, is a classification based on educational needs.

I am not, of course, in any way disputing the considerable educational needs of the slow learner, still less would I wish to be complacent in saying that these needs are adequately met in the present educational system. If provision is inadequate, however, this means only that authorities need to do better what they are doing already. In contrast, if a child is "discrepant", his needs are quite different. "Discrepant" children who display the dyslexic signs require, for practical purposes to be classified as a special group, identifiable by a word which makes clear that they are *handicapped*. They will be thoroughly unhappy and out of place in a class for slow learning children; and in this case it is not that the educational system should try to do better what it is doing already, but that it should set out to do something different, that is recognize dyslexia as a special category of disability and make provision for it.

If one allows that discrepancy between intelligence level and performance at reading and spelling is a necessary condition for saying that a child is dyslexic, the question then arises as to how large the discrepancy needs to be. Here it seems to me that the only relevant considerations are pragmatic ones. One must ask, Is the discrepancy large enough to be taken seriously? If it is, then to that extent the child is different and needs special attention, and the word "dyslexic" marks the difference.

On this showing the reasons for classifying a child as "dyslexic" are social and educational rather than physiological. Whatever the exact nature of the underlying physiological failure, the important manifestations socially and educationally are difficulty with reading and difficulty with spelling. It is therefore convenient to separate out as a special group those children who, because of constitutional limitations, require individual help in these two areas. In particular they need to be distinguished from children who are slow at *all* school subjects but who learn to read and even spell without all that much difficulty.

Where the discrepancy is not all that great it seems to me perfectly reasonable to say of a child that he is "very slightly dyslexic", or to say that one discovered a few signs of possible dyslexia which were not severe enough to be taken seriously. There are, of course, parallels in other fields: a person might have a very mild astigmatism, insufficiently severe to justify the wearing of glasses. In general, just because a particular handicap or illness can sometimes be very mild it does not follow that in the severe cases nothing needs to be done.

Indeed, in the case of dyslexia it seems to me most important that any handicap which exists should not be played down. It can be far more harmful, in my experience, to tell the parents not to worry when a dyslexic child is appreciably handicapped than to describe a child as dyslexic when his handicap is only minimal. An unnecessary diagnosis of dyslexia is likely to do little damage, since the child merely receives some extra tuition which he did not really need, whereas there is clear evidence that failure to recognize that a child is dyslexic (and hence needs special tuition) can be very costly in terms of frustration and under-achievement. Large numbers of parents have reported to me that they have been fobbed off with the facile statement, "Don't worry; he'll grow out of it" when they told the teacher that they suspected something was wrong. Underestimating the degree of handicap seems to me a far more serious error than over-estimating it.

(4) Finally there is the situation where there appears to be some kind of learning "block" even though reading and spelling are not too seriously affected.

Philip came to me at the age of 10 years 1 month. The Terman test showed him to be of average ability; his "reading age" on the Schonell word-recognition test came out as 9 years 4 months (93% of his chronological age) and his "spelling age" came out at exactly 9 years (90% of his chronological age). On its own this discrepancy would not perhaps be large enough to justify the claim that Philip was in any way unusual. He was referred, however, because of special problems with arithmetic. "What I find particularly unusual at his age" wrote Philip's headmaster, "is that he... lacks appreciation of order in numbers. For instance, in simple multiplication involving 3×8, he is perfectly liable to put down the 2 in the units column and carry the 4 into the tens column. I have used an abacus and virtually every other method to indicate tens and units to him, but nevertheless mistakes still recur."

Despite his relatively high score on the word-recognition and spelling tests, I discovered plenty of signs belonging in the "dyslexia" family. When I asked him to say "3-4-1-7" after me he said "3-1-4-7," and when I gave him three digits to say in reverse order he failed to get the order correct in two trials out of three (with, of course, different digits on each trial). This response is well outside normal limits for a 10-year old of average ability. There was continual confusion of b and d in his writing, for example "boll" for "doll," "barsing" for "dancing" and "binermite" for "dynamite." There were also other strange mistakes of a typically "dyslexic" kind: "prepterion" for "preparation" (later "prparlion"), "torw brigde" for "Tower Bridge," "wroy" for "worry," "Amecar" for "America," and "libtgh" for "light." He needed to use his fingers for simple calculation; he lost his place in saying his six-times and seven-times tables, and in trying to explain his arithmetical difficulties to me he said "All double numbers—I sometimes put them the wrong way round."

If one insists that no one can be classified as dyslexic unless there is an appreciable discrepancy between spelling attainment and intellectual level, one cannot logically apply the word dyslexic to Philip. The difficulties and mistakes, however, belong so clearly in the dyslexia family that such a conclusion would be absurd. A whole host of dyslexic signs were so clearly present that I had no hesitation in classing him as dyslexic (though I expressed surprise to his mother that he had learned to spell so successfully). On practical grounds, of course, there was no doubt whatever that he needed specialist help on an individual basis.

From a consideration of Philip's case it follows that considerable caution is needed in interpreting the results of large-scale surveys. If one has figures only for I.Q., reading age and spelling age, one cannot logically make any firm statement about the incidence or existence of dyslexia. Compared with James (see pp. 13 *seq.*) Philip was relatively less retarded at both reading and spelling, yet the other evidence points inescapably to dyslexia, whereas James seems, at most a decidedly marginal case.

I have also heard of children who were reported to have a "block" in handling numbers but to have no problem at all over reading or spelling. Although I have not examined any such children myself, I have no grounds for doubting the accuracy of such claims. There is no reason why there should not be variants within the dyslexic groups of disabilities, just as there are variants in the form taken by an illness or in different species of insect or plant. We cannot expect nature to arrange things in completely tidy groups for us and she certainly does not! There is no reason, therefore, why there should not be handicaps which are like dyslexia in some ways and unlike it in others.

One final complication requires mention. I have occasionally met or heard of children who showed dyslexic signs in addition to having some reasonably clear-cut medical condition, such as autism (see Glossary) or minimal brain damage. In the case of autistic children who show dyslexic signs one cannot exclude the possibility that the difficulties with reading and spelling have put the child under such pressure that autism, or lack of contact with reality, has been the result; but it is clearly hard in many cases to isolate cause and effect or to be sure of

81

the part played by contributory or "predisposing" factors. In the case of minimal brain damage, there are grounds for saying that the total picture is somewhat different from that of dyslexia. Although these children, like some dyslexic children, may have been late at walking and acquiring speech and may show signs of speech defects, clumsiness and poor motor control, unlike the dyslexic child they are weak at *abstract* reasoning and often show an inability to think except in very concrete terms. A brain-damaged 15-year old whom I met some years ago was able to pick out hammer, nail and pliers from a miscellaneous group of objects as "belonging together," and he then said to me, "You put the nail in with the hammer and pull it out with the pliers," but he had the utmost difficulty in coming up with the word "carpentry." More recently, when I asked a boy who had signs of minimal brain damage how "wood" and "coal" were alike, he insisted on telling me how they were different. The typical dyslexic child, however, can usually do this kind of test with little difficulty. Thus although the signs of minimal brain damage and the signs of dyslexia sometimes overlap, there seems to me to be a good case for keeping the two conditions separate.

I have tried in this chapter to show some of the reasons why in particular cases one may be unsure whether or not to call a person "dyslexic." Absence of factual information is one such reason, but there are in addition semantic problems, the answer to which depends on how one chooses to classify. Most of the dyslexic children whom

I have seen have in fact been clear-cut cases, but it is not impossible that from time to time one will come across children who are only mildly or marginally dyslexic, as well as other children whose diagnosis is complicated by the presence of additional factors, such as general slowness, autism or brain damage.

4

What Causes Dyslexia?

IT seems to me to be established beyond reasonable doubt that the difficulties which have been described in Chapters 1 and 2 are constitutional in origin. This does not mean, of course, that environmental influences play no part at all. If a dyslexic child is lucky enough to receive appropriate teaching at an early age, the ill-effects of his dyslexia can be minimized; and if his parents and his teachers are sympathetic and make clear that they understand his particular difficulties, he will be under much less strain. In that sense an adverse environment can contribute to the total difficulties, whereas a highly favourable one can lessen them; but this is not to say that the adverse environment is the main causal agency.

There are, of course, many kinds of handicap, for example lameness due to poliomyelitis, where sympathetic handling can play an important part but where the basic cause is constitutional. The same holds true in the case of dyslexia. Indeed, however much compensation there may be for its effects, it is important to realize that one is dealing with a child who has a constitutionally caused handicap.

Once a handicap is present there may, of course, be all kinds of further causal chains which lead to different results in different cases. Thus a child who is potentially dyslexic may be under appreciably less difficulty if the language which he has to write is a phonetically regular one—Welsh, for instance, as compared with English or French. Again, some children react to their disability by becoming discouraged, while others show extra determination to succeed. Similarly, pressures in the home and at school may contribute to the child's reactions in all kinds of ways. All such factors, however, must clearly be regarded as secondary: the basic causal explanation lies in some kind of defect in the mechanisms for perceiving and remembering.

The details of this defect are not known, and the amateur neurological speculations of some psychologists and educationalists often seem to me to be rather unprofitable. In particular those who suppose that there can be "faults" in the brain in much the same way as there are sometimes faults in an electrical system are perhaps guilty of oversimplification. In fact, if one part of the brain is damaged another part can sometimes take over some of the requisite functions, and even when a child or adult is known to have fairly gross brain damage, as in cases of aphasia (see Glossary), it is not easy to predict the extent to which he will be able to compensate or learn new skills. In the case of dyslexia the situation may well be even more problematic, and while I do not doubt that there *is* a neurological explanation for the dyslexic group of difficulties there are no good grounds for supposing that this explanation is a simple one.

The circumstantial evidence for a constitutional factor, however, is extremely strong. There are four main types

85

of consideration which are relevant here: (1) the fact that the condition runs in families, (2) the fact that it is more common in boys than in girls, (3) the fact that there is a similarity between the mistakes made by dyslexic children and those made by adult aphasic patients, and (4) the fact that there is no regular association between dyslexic difficulties and any particular environmental influence such as poor teaching.

In what follows I shall comment on these four points in turn.

1 : *The condition runs in families*

That the condition runs in families cannot seriously be doubted. Research reports from a variety of sources have been summarized by Critchley (1970, pp. 89 *seq.*; see Further Reading, p. 135, no. 1), who asserts that "We owe to genetics the most cogent single argument in support of the conception of a constitutional specific type of dyslexia identifiable among the miscellany of cases of poor readers." He cites, for instance, the work of Hallgren in Scandinavia, who claimed that, of 276 cases, 88% had reading problems in one or more relatives. Also, in twelve pairs of monozygotic (see Glossary) twins with dyslexia he reported a finding of 100% "concordance," that is to say, in all cases *both* twins had the difficulties.

It is always possible in this area to raise doubts about the quality of the evidence. Not all investigators have used precisely the same criteria for determining if a child is dyslexic, and quite apart from this, accurate evidence about other members of the family is not always easy to obtain; the information that "Uncle Jack was never a very good speller," is scant evidence on which to base a diagnosis of dyslexia! Even if one has a few reservations of this kind, however, the general conclusion that the condition sometimes runs in families seems to me to be established beyond reasonable doubt.

Our experience at Bangor confirms this point. Time and time again we have found that more than one member of a family has been affected. For example, a father gave me a description of his own difficulties which clearly showed that they were dyslexic in character, while his three sons were all found, on testing, to have similar difficulties, albeit only mildly in the case of two of them. In another case a mother, who was a mathematics graduate, reported regular difficulty over distinguishing left and right and actually made an error when required to repeat three digits reversed and her son, although extremely intelligent, showed all the typical dyslexic signs. On a number of occasions I have assessed two brothers both of whom were found to be dyslexic, and there have been times when I have described the difficulties of the dyslexic child to parents and they have immediately volunteered the information, "I think I have had similar difficulties myself."

Perhaps the most striking example in my own experience of familial incidence of dyslexia occurred in the case of Robert's relatives (cf. p. 38). Robert's uncle, a university physics lecturer, produced a record, dated 1938, showing he had been assessed at a child guidance clinic and found to be severely behindhand at reading and spelling despite an outstandingly high result on an intelligence test. Even now he cannot do simple subtraction without using his fingers as concrete aids and he is said to dislike strongly reading letters in manuscript! His son, Alex, Robert's cousin, who came to me at the age of $7\frac{1}{2}$, was found to have an I.Q. of 144 and all the same difficulties. When Alex and his parents recently visited the U.S.A. they met two second cousins, one aged 10, the other aged 8. The older was said to have had "considerable difficulty with spelling and reading earlier, but is now reported to have overcome the problems," while the younger was still "having considerable difficulty with spelling." Alex's mother told me that the great grandfather of these boys (who was, of course, also the great grand-father of Robert and Alex) had translated works from Russian into English, but had been very unhappy at school "because he had been unable to learn by rote"; this was confirmed by Robert's mother. All four of this man's sons were reported to be poor spellers; one of them, so I was told, "read very slowly because he made the tongue and lip movements of the words he was reading." Some of the evidence here is admittedly second or third hand, but there is no reason to doubt its basic reliability, and I myself have detailed evidence of Alex, Alex's father and Robert. In the case of this family it is, in my opinion, impossible to doubt the familial incidence of a disability. Any other explanation of difficulties occurring so frequently in such an obviously able family (even when the members were on different sides of the Atlantic!) would commit one to belief in a truly remarkable string of coincidences.

2 : *It is more common in boys than in girls*

The second line of evidence, which again suggests a genetic factor, is that the condition is appreciably more common in boys than in girls. Here, too, Critchley (*op. cit.*, p. 91) has marshalled the evidence. On the basis of nineteen different surveys between 1927 and 1968 he reaches the conclusion that the incidence is four times as common in males than in females.

Again our experience at Bangor confirms this. At the time of writing we had data on 185 established cases, of whom 145 were boys and 40 were girls. The ratio of boys to girls is thus about $3\frac{1}{2}$: 1.

As it stands, this evidence does not, of course, decisively exclude the possibility that social factors rather than genetic factors are responsible for the difference. Thus it could be argued that girls mature earlier than boys or that for a variety of reasons parents are more ready to seek help for a boy than for a girl. It seems to me far more likely, however, that a genetic factor is involved, since, even if these other factors play a part, it is hard to see how, on their own, they could explain an imbalance of this magnitude.

3 : *The mistakes are like those made by aphasic patients*

The similarity between the mistakes made by dyslexic children and those made by brain-damaged adults seems to me one which should certainly be taken seriously. It is hard to argue convincingly here, since the appeal is perhaps largely to the "feel" of particular cases; one is saying in effect, "This feels just like the kind of mistake which a brain-damaged adult would make." But we know for certain that brain damage in adults can sometimes result in difficulty in appreciating spatial and temporal relationships; and since mistakes made by a dyslexic child have the same "feel" (as in my experience they certainly do), it is surely correct to conclude that a constitutional factor is at work. One is right here, I think, to follow the lead of MacMeeken (1959, p. 27; see Further Reading, p. 136, no. 10) who says, "There can be no doubt whatever that we are in touch with a pattern of difficulty *aphasic* in type."

Critchley, too (*op. cit.*, pp. 73–4), though suitably cautious, is in no doubt about the similarities. "When spatial disabilities occur," he writes, "they recall those met with in adult patients with parietal lobe lesions, differing however in that they are manifesting themselves at an earlier age, and that they are less elaborate and less conspicuous. As in acquired parietal disease they are highly diverse in their nature." He goes on to describe some of the things that can happen in particular cases: "There may be a dimensional confusion so that elevation and plan are jumbled up in an odd manner. Even greater spatial defects may at times be shown when the dyslexic draws from memory a clock-face or a bicycle. Their efforts may be uncoordinated and even confused . . . The dyslexic child may mix up extra-corporeal spatial directions such as up and down, and more often still, left and right. Prepositions such as on, under, below, behind, beyond may be muddled. In attempting to write or to make arithmetical calculations, the child may set down the words and figures upon the paper in an irregular and even haphazard fashion. Figures and words are not placed under each other in correct alignment: the left-hand margins may be too narrow or too wide, and often they descend obliquely." Later he refers to children who show difficulties on the temporal side, and cites the case of a child who said "the day after yesterday . . . I mean the day before tomorrow," when he had meant to say "the day after tomorrow" (*ibid.*, p. 82).

In the case of dyslexic children it is arguable that one should think in terms of failure of development rather than in terms of acquired injury. This is the hypothesis of "maturational lag." On this showing a dyslexic child is *late* in developing the mechanisms needed for spelling, left-right discrimination, and so on. It seems to me doubtful, however, if lateness is all that is involved. There are doubtless many adults who have achieved success despite their dyslexia; but, to judge from those with whom I have talked, it seems to me incorrect to say simply that they have "grown out of" their dyslexia in the way in which a child who is late at walking may "grow out of it" and walk quite normally later in life. That they have learned to live with their dyslexia is not in dispute, nor is it in dispute that they may have learned all kinds of ingenious ways of compensating for their disability or covering it up. My suspicion, however—based admittedly on only a small number of cases—is that there are some tasks, such as saying digits in reverse order or repeating the months of the year backwards, which even dyslexic adults still find difficult; and in that case one is wrong to think simply of late development, but one should think rather of a handicap which will continue to be present even though the person discovers or is taught ways of minimizing its effects.

A further point which needs to be considered is that some dyslexic children show evidence of minimal brain dysfunction: they are reported as having been late at walking and talking and are sometimes found to have mild speech defects and to display clumsiness and poor motor control despite ability to reason in the abstract (cf. p. 82). In these cases it is reasonable to suppose that the same failure—whatever its precise nature—accounts both for these "soft neurological signs" and for the difficulties in reading, spelling and temporal and spatial orientation; and it is not impossible that they are due to a somewhat more diffuse group of faults than those which are present in the more "pure" and less complicated types of dyslexia. In general it seems to me that in this area we must face the fact that the difficulties are somewhat varied; certainly up till the present no very clear sub-categories within the group of dyslexic children have emerged.

4: *Dyslexia is not regularly associated with any one feature in the environment*

No alternative hypothesis, involving environmental as opposed to constitutional factors, seems at all plausible. If emotional maladjustment were the main factor, this would not explain the occurrence of dyslexic difficulties in those children who were not emotionally maladjusted. If poor teaching were the main factor, one would expect dyslexia to occur among several children who had attended the same class, and this plainly does not happen. If parental pressure were the main factor, this would not explain the variety of reactions displayed by parents to their child's difficulties; still less would it explain why children who were subjected to such pressures always responded by failing in the same specific, limited areas.

Certainly if one *treats* the disability as constitutional, the reaction of both parents and children is that this makes sense. In many of the families whom I myself have seen, there has been complete bewilderment over the child's difficulties; and when I have indicated some of the manifestations of dyslexia (such as difficulty over remembering tables and difficulty over spatial and temporal sequencing), the reaction has almost invariably been one of relief that at last an explanation is being offered which accounts both for the child's obvious ability and for his failure in certain areas. Evidence based on the study of parents' and children's reactions is admittedly not conclusive on its own, but when considered in conjunction with other evidence it strengthens one's belief that these dyslexic difficulties are constitutionally caused.

Some writers have called attention to an association between dyslexia and unusual patterns of handedness and eye-dominance. In particular they have pointed out that dyslexic children have a greater tendency to be "cross-lateral," in the sense of being right-handed and left-eyed or left-handed and right-eyed. It has also been suggested that in some cases there is poorly developed cerebral dominance: in other words the child is neither clearly right-handed nor clearly left-handed.

It seems to me that speculations in this area should be treated with a certain amount of caution. To begin with, many researches have shown that plenty of those with dyslexia are straightforwardly right-handed and right-eyed and, although there is some evidence that cross-laterality is more common among dyslexic children than among non-dyslexic children, any suggestion of a direct causal relationship remains unproven. Also such a hypothesis would, at best, account only for those cases of dyslexia where there *was* cross-laterality, and one would be in the uncomfortable position of having to find a different explanation for dyslexia where there was *no* cross-laterality. In my experience cross-laterality is of no special use even as a diagnostic sign, since there are plenty of people who are cross-lateral without being dyslexic and plenty of people who are dyslexic without being cross-lateral. Even though there are grounds for saying that more dyslexic children have unusual handedness patterns or that more are cross-lateral than one would expect in the normal population, the significance of this association is very hard to interpret.

One final point about causation needs to be mentioned. There is perhaps a tendency in the case of dyslexia to overestimate the importance of finding out what causes it.

There are many situations where knowledge of the cause provides the key for appropriate treatment. Most of the standard cases of what we call "disease" are of this kind: one kills off the virus, remedies the vitamin deficiency, and so on. Dyslexia, however, is somewhat different. It is not something which one "catches," like a skin infection. Indeed it is perhaps misleading even to say that someone has "got" dyslexia as one might say that he had "got" measles. A more accurate formulation, I think, is to describe dyslexia not as a disease but as a "disability" or "handicap."

From the treatment point of view it is important to appreciate that the cause is constitutional, since this entails that we cannot attribute the condition to such factors as parental neuroticism or poor teaching. The precise details, however, are not of major importance for the teacher. This is because one does not attempt to "cure" dyslexia by rectifying whatever the constitutional fault may be; one tries to alleviate a handicap by appropriate teaching.

Similarly, while it may be of considerable theoretical interest if future research shows differences in E.E.G. records (see Glossary) between dyslexic children and controls, as far as the practical problems of the teacher are concerned such findings seem unlikely to be of any help. The question which needs to be asked of a teaching method is, Does it work? In general it seems to me more important, at least in our present state of knowledge, that time and effort should be spent on the discovery of improved teaching techniques than that time and effort should be spent on research into causation.

Perhaps one of the reasons why there has been argument and controversy over dyslexia is that it lies uncomfortably on the boundary between medicine and education; and indeed some of the polemics which I have read have seemed to me rather like petty disputes over "ownership." As I see the situation, dyslexia is a medical matter in its origin and an educational matter as regards treatment. Both medical and educational considerations are therefore important for its understanding, and it is most desirable that suitable attention should be paid to both.

5

Problems of Screening

THE magnitude of the dyslexia problem is still far from
clear. As shown in Chapters 2 and 3, there is no difficulty
in picking out the obvious cases; but there may be children whose handicap is only marginal and perhaps others
who, because of their constitutional make-up, were at
risk but have learned to cope more or less adequately.
Any attempt to specify what percentage of the school
population is dyslexic will of necessity involve a somewhat arbitrary cut-off point. What seems to me important
is a screening system which picks out those whose need is
greatest.

In most areas at the present time the discovery of
dyslexic children seems often to be left to individual
initiative. Sometimes this initiative may come from a
medical officer, sometimes from a psychologist, sometimes
from a teacher, sometimes from a parent. It is true that
in many counties reading tests are carried out on all
children aged 7 and upwards. The objection to this procedure, however, is that it will necessarily reveal only an
amorphous mass of poor readers of all kinds. Although
this group may well contain children who are dyslexic,
many of the brighter dyslexic children may escape this
particular net, since their reading may not be all that far
behind the norm for their age, even though their

97

intelligence level on a test which does not require much reading may be very high. Such children may, of course, be very unhappy in school if suitable provision is not made for them.

I have come across situations where there is a serious failure of communication between medical and educational authorities. Indeed on one occasion I received a request from a medical authority (not in my own area, be it said) to assess a boy who might be dyslexic—only to have this request countermanded by someone who worked for the same authority on the educational side! Adequate liaison seems essential; and in a particular case it may be necessary to eliminate certain handicaps which are primarily of medical concern, such as poor eyesight, poor hearing and minimal brain damage, before the correct educational measures can start. As we have seen (p. 95–6), dyslexia is not a problem for doctors only, nor for teachers only—it is a problem for both.

One possibility* is that every 9-year old should be given a piece of free composition. It is fair to assume that those who manage adequately have no particular spelling problem, while those who do not can be investigated further. This, however, is only a beginning. One has to consider the whole pattern of symptoms, as described in Chapter 2. Teachers' reports may be very useful, and one possible procedure is to ask the teacher to consider the various items given in Appendix II (pp. 127–32) and see if they apply to a particular child. It is unfortunate when large-scale and expensive surveys are conducted in

* I owe this suggestion to Miss G. C. Cotterell, Remedial Advisory Teacher to the Suffolk School Psychological Service.

such a way that they do not distinguish dyslexic children from other children whose needs are quite different. As we have seen already in the cases of James and Philip (p. 73 *seq.*, 79 *seq.*), two children whose degree of retardation is the same if one judges by the results of intelligence and attainment tests may in fact have needs which are entirely different.

The fact that things are at present often left to individual initiative is particularly regrettable in that large numbers of children do not receive the help that they need. A further unfortunate result is that, because the initiative is often taken by the parents, some people have been disposed to sneer that dyslexia is a "disease of the middle classes." This remark seems to me both uninformed and uncharitable. Dyslexia should in any case be recognized not as a disease but rather as a handicap (cf. pp. 94–5) and my experience in the North Wales area leaves me in no doubt at all that this handicap can occur in children of all kinds of social background. Admittedly it is the parents with a special concern for education who are most likely to take the initiative in pressing that something be done; and indeed in this book I have for the most part quoted evidence based on discussions with the more articulate parents. To suppose, however, that dyslexia is limited to the children of such parents is palpably absurd. The correct procedure, it seems to me, is not to indulge in sneers about the middle classes (who in any case are not the only section of the population to care about literacy), but to make methods of screening more effective and thus ensure that no dyslexic child is overlooked whatever his background.

6

Dyslexia and Morale

DYSLEXIC children react to their disability in a variety of different ways. I have met a few who were somewhat happy-go-lucky, or at least managed to seem so, but the majority, in my experience, have undergone appreciable hardship, particularly if they had been at school for a number of years before their disability was recognized and explained to them.

It does not take long, I believe, for an intelligent dyslexic child in his early days at school to realize that he is different from his classmates. He may not know exactly what is wrong, but almost every lesson is likely to show up the differences. Even at a young age he may discover that other children can please the teacher by making the right noise when shown a piece of paper or a blackboard with what is to him a blur of complex marks on it, and can please her again by writing the right letters in the right order when asked to spell something. He may indeed discover that if these marks on paper are accompanied by a picture (as happens in most books designed for young children) he can gain some approval by describing the picture and ignoring the marks themselves, although his classmates, it seems, can say the correct words even when no picture is present. As a result of his failure he may be branded as "lazy" or "stupid," and may indeed come to believe this. It therefore seems to me particularly important that, as soon as his dyslexia is recognized, the precise nature of his difficulties should be explained to him. To pretend that they do not exist is likely only to increase his fears and uncertainties.

The fact that a child has failed in particular areas may result in some cases in a more general sense of failure. Because he is no good at certain reading and spelling tasks, it is easy for him to assume that he is no good at anything. If he has a clear understanding of where his special weaknesses lie, he will be able to make a clear distinction between these weaknesses and other things which he can do perfectly well. Above all, if he has continuous experience of success in some areas, his difficulties in other areas will be less of a worry to him.

There is no need for him to become frightened of words as such. He is capable of deriving real enjoyment if stories or poetry are read to him, and there is no reason why he should not enjoy such "word games" as riddles, puns, jokes and repartee when given orally, even though it may be too difficult for him to understand what is involved if he is dependent on books and magazines.

Several people have suggested (rightly, in my opinion) that dyslexic children are often young for their age. It follows from this that a certain amount of extra "mothering" may be very helpful to them; and it is a pity that some popular magazines and even, perhaps, some professional counsellors have tended to foster a climate of opinion in which the "over-fussy" mother is adversely criticized.

The Dyslexic Child

Here, by way of illustration, is a brief sketch of a dyslexic boy whose mother had the courage to back her own judgment against that of her many advisers.

Michael first came to me at the age of $8\frac{1}{2}$. His mother, who was separated from her husband, had been left to care both for Michael and for his elder sister who was also dyslexic. Well-wishers had told her that the absence of a father was responsible for her children's educational difficulties—an attitude no less cruel for being predictable. Michael was reported as being in the very superior range of intelligence, but when I tested his reading and spelling I found he had a "reading age" of $5\frac{3}{4}$ and a "spelling age" of $6\frac{1}{2}$. He wrote "doll" as "boll" and "cap" as "caq"; "land" was written as "lad" and "cold" as "cod." When asked to say the months of the year he replied "I don't know," and, after prompting, said "February, August, December, November." Then, after correctly repeating his four-times table as far as $7 \times 4 = 28$, he said "Where have I got to? I get mixed up."

After some abortive attempts to find a suitable school, his mother gave up the struggle and kept him at home, doing the teaching herself. I had given her some guidance as to the kind of thing needed with a dyslexic child. I became convinced—as she was—that to place a bright and sensitive dyslexic boy in the kind of day-school which existed near her home was to put him in an impossible situation. Her well-wishers told her how stupid and over-protective she was being, but she backed her own judgment against theirs.

When I retested Michael eighteen months later his "reading age" had gone up by 2 years and 5 months and even his "spelling age" (on a test which is unsuitable and difficult for dyslexic children), had gone up by 1 year and 4 months. At this stage, at the age of 10, he was becoming ready to go to an ordinary school. Fortunately a suitable one has been found where dyslexia is recognized and where there is a happy "family" atmosphere. I myself believe that his mother was entirely right to have kept him at home in the meantime.

In general it may often be the case that the parents of a dyslexic child are sensitive to his needs in a way that outsiders cannot be. Adverse criticisms, whether spoken or implied, of parental "over-fussiness" may sometimes be quite misguided.

Finally, it is important to remember the pressures which are imposed on the dyslexic child by the educational system. There is a premium on literacy, and in most schools most of the time there is, rightly or wrongly, an atmosphere of competitiveness. If a dyslexic child is judged by normal standards of "success" and "failure," he is bound to feel insecure, inadequate, incompetent. What is required is an adjustment of standards to take account of what he can and cannot easily do. Expecting nothing of a dyslexic child violates his self-respect as much as expecting everything of him. What is necessary is that all who come into contact with him should be aware both of his strengths and of his limitations.

7

Organizing the Teaching

THIS chapter is not concerned with teaching methods as such, since I have discussed these elsewhere (see references 11 and 12, p. 136). It may be helpful, however, if I offer some comments on the various administrative problems associated with teaching. I shall consider in particular the question of how to find the most suitable teacher and the question of the most suitable time and place for the lessons.

At the time of writing (though this may not hold in the future) one cannot, I think, be over-particular as to whether the proposed teacher has the appropriate paper qualifications. A willingness to understand the child's difficulties is far more important.

I have occasionally met qualified teachers who give the impression that they think they "know all the answers." They report that they have never failed to teach a child to read (which may in fact be true, though I cannot believe that it is true in the case of teaching to spell), and if they believe in dyslexia at all one gets the impression that they do not take seriously the idea that the child is dyslexic. This kind of teacher is best avoided.

To take the child's dyslexia seriously is to recognize that he has a disability or handicap. Such recognition is perfectly possible for those who have had little or no teaching experience. If the person is flexible in his approach, willing to learn, and willing to profit from his mistakes, he may well be more effective than those who on paper are better qualified. By "he" I mean, of course, "he or she", for many successful teachers of dyslexic children have in fact been women. Whether to opt for a man or woman teacher will depend on the circumstances of each case. I have met many children of all ages who were ready and willing to learn from either.

Perhaps surprisingly, I have not found age to be a serious obstacle. Those who have retired from full-time active teaching or work at colleges of education may often be glad to do part-time work with dyslexic children, and I have known several cases where such people have been extremely successful. In the case of older and more intelligent dyslexic children it is perhaps desirable that the teacher should be a gratitude or at least someone who can provide suitable intellectual stimulation.

The ideal situation is one in which the dyslexic child receives 20–25 minutes' tuition per day four or five times a week. In practice, because of difficulties over travelling, this is not always possible. As an absolute minimum one must insist on once weekly lessons, and if they are as infrequent as this it is very desirable that some member of the child's family, or perhaps a trainee teacher, should provide "revision" periods between lessons. Also there may be unavoidable breaks—because of half-term, illness, and so on—and if the once-weekly session itself becomes eroded, the stage may be reached where lack of progress becomes extremely frustrating. A teacher unfamiliar with dyslexia may underestimate the amount of forgetting which occurs.

Teachers should also be alerted to the possibility that the child needs special help with arithmetic as well as with reading and spelling.

The actual administration of the remedial teaching requires thought. There are many advantages if it is done within the precincts of the child's school: much time is saved, and teaching aids and equipment are readily available. More important, however, is the question of the child's morale. It is no kindness, it seems to me, simply to require a dyslexic child to do "special reading" or "special spelling," as one might, for instance, require a child who was weak at geography to do "special geography." A dyslexic child, as I have continually pointed out has a *disability*, and he needs to know this. Whether or not he keeps this knowledge to himself or shares it publicly is up to him, but there is a world of difference between "not being very good at reading or spelling"—a discouraging condition which creates a sense of failure—and being dyslexic, since the latter involves a challenge to overcome limitations which are known not to be his fault. It is important, therefore, that the remedial services should be so organized that the special nature of the disability is made clear. This can be achieved either by taking the child out of school to a special venue or by arranging for him to go to a special room in the school buildings where help for dyslexic children is regularly given. There is no doubt at all, in my opinion, that most children are helped if one "makes a thing" of their dyslexia rather than plays it down; and it seems to me important that this point should be reflected in the way in which the facilities for remedial teaching are planned.

It is also important that the time when the remedial lessons are fixed should be convenient for both teacher and child. The amount of concentration needed is such that no teacher can possibly be expected to take more than three 55-minute sessions without a break; and from the child's point of view it is most important that the lesson should not clash with his favourite out-of-school activity—whether football, swimming, canoeing or whatever it may be. It is also most desirable that the lessons should be fixed early in the day; at four o'clock in the afternoon or later one often sees signs of weariness such as stifled yawns!

In some cases it is necessary for the teaching to be done completely outside the school. Even then, it is important that the lessons should be held during school hours: after school the child is tired, and on a Saturday morning he may be longing to go off on a bicycle ride with his friends or join in some family activity. A successful lesson is likely to be very hard work, and the conditions need to be right if the child is to give of his best. It is also very desirable that the person doing the teaching should keep in close touch with the school.

In some cases considerable help can be given by the child's parents. As I have indicated already p. 101), I think it is important that one should forget some of the things which one reads in the press and in educational books about "problem parents." I have met a number of families where the mother has successfully embarked on a remedial programme, as happened in the cases of

Henry (pp. 16 *seq.*) and Michael (pp. 102–3), and on one
occasion the teaching was done by the father. Clearly
the position will vary from one family to another, but it
seems to me that in many families the parents can be of
enormous help.

Finally, it remains to be considered whether there are
any basic principles which all teachers of dyslexic
children need to know. Personally I believe that there are,
though perhaps not everyone would share this view.

I think it likely that one of the basic difficulties with
many, if not all, dyslexic children is that the amount of
material which they can absorb in a given time is severely
limited. This means that, even though they may sometimes correctly respond to longer words (of six or seven
letters or more), the details of these words almost certainly
escape them. As a result, attempts to spell such words
will very often be unsuccessful. It therefore seems
desirable, at least in the majority of cases, to use an
out-and-out phonic approach. One needs to start, in
other words, by showing the child how each letter re-
presents its own distinctive sound. Later he can be shown
how different combinations of letters sometimes make the
same sound, for instance that "ea" and "ee" both make
the long e-sound, as in "keen," but this should not be
introduced too early. What is important is that he should
acquire the habit of looking at the *details* of a word and
should be shown how the particular letter-sounds combine
to make the word. Phonetically irregular words should
therefore not be introduced too early, and when the time
comes for introducing them the fact that they are

irregular should be made clear. Such a teaching programme must necessarily be structured and cumulative: words should be specially chosen so as to illustrate the general principle which the child is being asked to learn (and many dyslexic children, of course, are very quick at learning general principles), while harder combinations of letters should not be introduced until the easier ones have been mastered.

In choosing a teacher, therefore, it is very desirable to find someone who is willing to think about problems of reading and spelling in this kind of way. Perhaps the greatest virtues in this area are humility and a dogged determination. If a teacher says to me, "I have never yet failed to teach a child to read," I am likely to feel uneasiness and doubt. In contrast, I was very happy, not long ago, to talk with a teacher who had had wide experience with some very severely dyslexic children: she made no facile boasts of her successes, which I knew were many, but said simply, "I never like being beaten."

8

The Dyslexic Child Grows Up

I WANT, in this final chapter, to give some indication as to what are reasonable objectives for a dyslexic child at different ages. Clearly no unqualified answers are possible, since individuals differ in all kinds of ways, but even rough and approximate guidelines may be better than none at all.

Our present experience suggests that, if a child of average general ability is found to be dyslexic, special teaching in reading and spelling should start when he is aged around $7\frac{1}{2}$ years old. If he receives two (or even three) years of such teaching there is a reasonable chance that, by the time he reaches the secondary school stage at age 11, his reading level will be not far short of the norm for his age. Spelling may inevitably be somewhat behind, but with suitable teaching the gap need not be all that wide. As has been indicated already, his arithmetic may need special help, too. If by the age of 9 or 10 he is brought to the stage where he can read books for pleasure and is no longer put off by them, one has good grounds for satisfaction.

As pointed out in Chapter 2 (p. 53), it is perhaps wise not to attach too much weight to an I.Q. figure. On the other hand it would, I think, be wrong to attach no weight to it at all. Given the educational system as it is at present, an I.Q. figure gives some kind of indication of whether a child is likely to succeed in academic subjects. Even in the case of a dyslexic child the figure is still a rough guide, despite the fact that the situation is complicated by a larger number of unknowns. It is, I think, essential to take into account not the "composite" I.Q. figure but rather the child's performance on those items which present no special difficulty for dyslexic children, but one must also remember that for the dyslexic child there are extra difficulties to be overcome. If the I.Q. figure is no more than average, I do not say that courses with an academic bias are impossible (I question the wisdom of saying that anything in the educational field is impossible until one has explored many different methods over a long period of time), but at least they are likely to be very difficult. Also the less intelligent dyslexic children will be less able to show ingenuity in compensating for their weaknesses. With an I.Q. figure of, say, 115 and upwards, however, there seems to me every case for giving a dyslexic child the chance to do academic courses, provided one does not press him to continue with them if they are too much of an effort and provided one does not expect too much too soon. In my experience many bright dyslexic children are glad to do academic work, and when the nature of their handicap has been explained to them many of them are perfectly willing to make the extra effort.

With older dyslexic children and dyslexic adults a test which I have found useful is the Advanced Matrices by J. C. Raven (see p. 125). It does not call for reading, memorizing or acquired knowledge. What is needed is that the person taking the test should make a series of complex deductions, on the basis of which he has to pick out the correct pattern, from a choice of eight, for completing a matrix. I have known many dyslexic adolescents who have scored very highly on this test, and there seems to me a good case for encouraging those who are successful to proceed with academic-type courses.

I have met quite a number of dyslexic children who were gifted at art and a small number—not, of course, the clumsy ones—who were gifted at ballet. Some, too, have been promising musicians, though in that case they should be warned not to be too discouraged if in the early stages reading notes from a musical stave presents some difficulty. A taste of success in *any* field, whether in art, music, sport or elsewhere, is likely to give a much-needed boost to morale, and it is very desirable that a dyslexic child should be given the opportunity to embark upon these activities if he so wishes.

It is not unusual for those with dyslexia to be "behind the clock" in passing examinations. To obtain passes at 'O' level at age 17 and above is by no means uncommon, while those who go on to 'A' level may be aged 20 or more before they are successful.

It is quite possible for a gifted dyslexic child eventually to reach university, and my experience is that those who have won through to this extent against the educational system are those of high stability and determination. The evidence suggests that such people may still be slower readers than their non-dyslexic colleagues and hence take a longer time to cover assignments, carry out a survey of relevant literature and so on. There is no doubt at all, however, that it is possible for those with dyslexia to achieve real distinction. I know of several successful doctors who have been dyslexic, of a highly successful actress, and of a university lecturer in English. There is, too, Alex's father (p. 87–8) who is a university lecturer in physics. The people concerned were, I am sure, of very high ability, but success at this level is certainly not impossible.

The examination system is unfortunately quite a hazard. Under stress a person with dyslexia may lose some of the skills which he has acquired; he may misread a question, for instance, or go "off the rails" in other ways, and what he finally puts down on paper may be a very inadequate reflection of what he actually knows. By now, however, most examining boards have expressed willingness to make allowance for dyslexic candidates: some permit extra time; some arrange for rereading for scripts, and at least one permits the services of an amanuensis.

More needs to be done, however, in my opinion, by way of persuading society not to impose unnecessary obstacles. For entry to training in some areas, for example, it is still customary to insist on a pass at 'O' level English; and this is something which many dyslexic children find difficult to achieve (cf. the case of Robert, p. 36 *seq.*). What is important here is that acceptance for a particular job or course of training should depend only on qualifications that are *relevant*. Clearly, for example, a certain level of proficiency in reading is necessary for a nurse, a postman, a storekeeper, etc., and it is quite reasonable to turn down any applicants, whether dyslexic or not, who fail to read at the required level. What is not reasonable is to require traditional standards of literacy without detailed consideration of the needs of a particular job; a dyslexic person who fails to reach these standards may in fact be able to do the job in question perfectly well.

There are perhaps certain occupations which are particularly unsuitable for anyone with dyslexia, or at least anyone whose dyslexia has been of an appreciable degree of severity—secretarial work, for instance, or work involving written French. In both cases the time and effort involved in consulting dictionaries, checking spellings, and so on would be very large indeed, and it would be unrealistic to expect any high degree of proficiency.

For most occupations, however, the main consideration must of course be what the person wants. The extent of the handicap will vary from one individual to another, and if someone aware of his handicap and aware of the demands of a particular job and of the training needed to qualify for that job chooses to make it his objective, then in my view it would not normally be right to try to dissuade him.

Here, to finish, are four further case studies. They are presented as an indication of the kinds of thing which can happen to a dyslexic child during adolescence and early adulthood.

Pamela

Pamela came to me at the age of 17. Her father, a doctor, wrote to me as follows: "We would very much appreciate [an appointment] as Pamela is much distressed at her inability to spell and the fact that she has failed English Language 'O' level twice."

When I gave her the Terman intelligence test I found that she had an I.Q. of 132, and her result included passes at the top grade of "superior adult." Yet her school books included some misspellings of what might seem to be easy words, such as "surtain" for "certain," "fearce" for "fierce," and "squesed" for "squeezed." In the Schonell test, which she did for me, her mistakes included "finacial" for "financial," "pliminary" for preliminary," "garentue" for "guarantee," and "irristable" for "irresistable." She spoke cheerfully, though not flatteringly, of teachers who "each try their little ways" of teaching her to spell, for example by setting her to learn ten words a day. She said, however, that her mother's phonic approach, unlike other methods, had been of help and that in addition she had evolved her own techniques: "A piece of cake is like a pie, so it is p-i-e, and peace—quiet —is the other one."

She reported that she sometimes made mistakes in arithmetic: "I might see 69 and write it as 96—I'd write it correctly and say it wrong . . . I always have to say it to check I've got it the right way round" (this is my record of what she said, but I suspect that even here she has somehow confused what she meant to say). "At one stage I used only the words I knew how to spell, but now I think 'Oh blow!' to them—they can correct the spelling themselves! . . . They say you must check it, but this is hopeless. I don't know how to spell it, so I can't."

Her original plan had been to train as a dental techni-
cian, but when she realized that her weak spelling was not
just the result of stupidity she was encouraged to take
'A' levels at a technical college. I do not know if she has
been successful, but on the evidence one can clearly rate
her chances highly.

Oliver

Oliver first came to me at the age of $15\frac{1}{2}$. His mother had
written to me as follows: "Though his reading ability
appears quite normal, he has always had more than the
average difficulty with spelling. Though this has improved
he is extremely handicapped by this problem. He has
had extra help both at school and at home without much
real success. Oliver is now most concerned himself and is
prepared to cooperate with any advice given."

When I gave him the Terman intelligence test I came
to realize what an enormous variety of different skills are
required to produce the correct answers. Some of these
skills Oliver possessed; but with others there appeared to
be some "block" or "handicap," as a result of which he
had to resort to roundabout methods which sometimes
enabled him to reach the right answers but which carried
considerable risk of error. Even within the same test item
some of the component skills presented him with no
difficulty while others left him struggling. For example.
there is one item in the Terman test which runs as
follows: "This time you have to bring back exactly 13
pints of water. You have a 9-pint can and a 4-pint can.
Show me how you can measure out exactly 13 pints of

water using nothing but these two cans and not guessing at the amount. You should begin by filling the 9-pint can first . . ." This item is difficult for many people because it calls for the ability to appreciate certain number-relationships and to select the relevant ones. Now Oliver had the special difficulty with arithmetic described on p. 64: he just did not know at a glance—as a non-dyslexic boy of his age and ability would have known—that $9 + 4 = 13$: for him that was the most difficult part of the test! The instruction book says that the subject should not use pencil or paper, but I decided to depart from this rule. After various pencil jottings he was able to decide that $9 + 4 = 13$, and with this information available he solved the "difficult" part of the problem instantaneously! Similarly he needed his own special diagrams to work out the answer to the question, "Which way would you have to face so that your left hand would be towards the east?" and in the end he was successful in a wide variety of items of this kind.

In general, although I was left with the impression that in many ways he was extremely bright, I found his Terman record impossible to score, since it was a patchwork of remarkable successes (including two passes at the most difficult section of all) and surprising failures, or, more strictly, failures which would have been surprising in a non-dyslexic boy of his ability.

On the Schonell word-recognition test he correctly read 73 out of the 100 words (which gives him a "reading age" at the 12-year level), while his "spelling age" came out at around $10\frac{1}{2}$. The following were some of the spelling mistakes which I noticed in his schoolbooks: "mtoity" for "majority," "argee" for "agree," "Tade uinions" for "trade unions," "temdos" for "tremendous," "fariself" for "for itself," and "pash" (with the letter r added between the s and h) for "parish," and "gaintic" for "gigantic." I noticed a comment to the effect that his spelling was "disgraceful," and I found that during the course of writing out the word "problems" 25 times (a technique which I do not advocate) his seventeenth attempt was "prodlems."

When asked to point to the left side of my body as I sat opposite him, he actually swivelled round in his seat before producing the correct answer. He failed to repeat the words "preliminary" and "statistics" correctly; he produced the right answers in the digits reversed test but only after long delay, during which he seemed to be mentally "writing" the digits in forward order on the paper in front of him. He failed in his first attempt to say the months of the year. He also had special difficulty in appreciating that two words rhyme. It seemed, for instance, as though he could tell that "head" and "red" rhymed only by spelling them out and noting the similarities between the last few letters. (I have met this difficulty occasionally in dyslexic children but it is too infrequent to include in a list of diagnostic signs.)

His mother explained that he wanted to be a civil engineer and asked if this was "right out of the question." I said that I did not know and that they would have to play the situation "by ear." I emphasized to both of them the remarkable skill and determination which Oliver had shown in learning to compensate for his disability and gave him every encouragement to continue with these efforts. His mother told me later that his comment after his interview was, "At last someone understands."

When I saw him again at the age of 17 I gave him the Advanced Matrices test (see p. 125) and his score came out at exactly the average figure given for university students.

Meanwhile he had made various attempts at "O" levels, with passes, over two years, at chemistry, history, geography, maths, physics and biology. His grades ranged from 6 to 3. His three attempts to take "O" level English resulted, successively, in grades 8, 9, and 7. My latest information is that he has left school and been accepted on a technical course leading to the Ordinary National Diploma, with the chance of later acceptance for the Higher National Diploma.

Life has certainly not been easy for Oliver. Indeed, one of his problems when he started his technical training was whether to explain his dyslexic difficulties to the course organizer. My personal view is that if one explains things to people they are likely to be sympathetic, but this is clearly something which Oliver must decide for himself. It is not impossible that he will make a further attempt at "O" level English, though this will depend on his eventual objectives. Clearly his difficulties with spelling and calculation are likely to remain as handicaps, but he may well achieve a great deal in spite of them. In a recent letter to me his mother spoke of his "determination to succeed" and ended by saying "He has come to terms with his problem and I am delighted."

The Dyslexic Child

Case 3: Andrew

Andrew was 18½-years old when he came to see me. His "reading age" came out as 12½ and his "spelling age" as just under 9 (the maximum possible reading and spelling age for an adult being 15). Yet on the basis of intelligence tests it was clear that this relatively poor performance was not the result of general slowness, and when I checked I found some clear dyslexic signs: he had to stand to turn his own body round before saying which was the left side of my body as I sat opposite him, he failed to repeat the polysyllabic words "preliminary" and "anemone;" he failed to repeat "four digits reversed" correctly (a task set to 9-year olds on the Terman test), he became confused in saying the months of the year, and said that when he counted he sometimes had to use his fingers. I saw him on 3rd August and when I asked if he knew today's date he said: "On the news it said 3rd May . . . oh, it's August . . . It's Wednesday; at least I hope it is. No, it's Tuesday—Thursday, rather."

Spelling mistakes included: "dughier" for "daughter," "egde" for "edge," "xpens" for "expense," "siret" for "street" and "prylmanarey for "preliminary." A school report said that if Andrew had more confidence his work would improve, and another report said that he "lacks effort." One teached had written, "In his last English homework he spelled 'tired' wrongly in one sentence and later spelled it correctly. Points to carelessness or lack of concentration."

Andrew's father could not work because of ill health, and his parents were of very restricted means. Owing to sympathetic help from the Department of Employment and Productivity, however, it was possible to finance some training at a special school where his dyslexia was understood. I saw some of the reports from the school, which were suitably encouraging without giving false reassurance, and every opportunity was taken to commend him for the things which he had done well. At present he is learning to be a chef, and I have every hope that he will be successful.

Phyllis

Finally, here is an account of Phyllis, who, like many dyslexic children, had an enormous struggle in the early stages.

She first came to me at the age of 10. Her I.Q. on the Terman test came out as 131, which is in the superior range, but her "reading age" was 9½ and her "spelling age" around 8½—far below what might be expected from a girl of that ability.

This is a sample of spelling, supplied by her mother: "Wlter rolgh was a yound menn woust to rob sponsch treasure shreps and he was a grote fo [crossed out] fat [crossed out and t altered to v] fovout of the Quen and he bunnt the fleat of sbne in the horbor, and he co [crossed out] cone book and said he hod bur the kens of spoin bred".

She had recently been given a "junior intelligence test" which contained a large number of written instructions. This was, of course, quite unsuitable in her case because of the time required for actual reading; and I noticed that when the written question was "A book in which the meanings of words are found" she had written "Becniory," which had been marked as wrong. A school report from a few years earlier said that she often wrote numerals the wrong way round, and a later report spoke of "extreme slowness and lack of drive." Another report said, "I feel Phyllis has much more ability than application . . . I am still waiting and hoping that Phyllis will really wake up."

Her parents were very much aware of her difficulties and she received special lessons from a teacher during the next year. "She is improving steadily" said her mother in a letter to me eight months later, "and is now half way through *The Borrowers* . . . Her spelling is not so bizarre and obviously shows signs of improvement; she can now spell words like 'once' correctly, although 'are' and 'out' still give trouble."

After a change of school at age eleven, she transferred at the age of $15\frac{1}{2}$ to a grammar school, where she later prepared to take "O" levels. When I saw her at age 16 her "reading age" was over 12 and her "spelling age" was about $10\frac{1}{2}$. She said that she was particularly keen to do science subjects and hoped eventually to read for a degree in medicine. Needless to say, I had no hesitation in supplying her with the appropriate certificate for presentation to her examining board.

She said that she still confused the letters a and o and occasionally made "silly mistakes" in maths. She had given up French because of the difficulty with the spelling. Her parents showed me a recent letter home, from which the following is extracted: ". . . as you know I was hoving trouble with the rector and I told him that I was worde blinde ond it tuoke a longe time to make him to make him there is sush a thing I think I convinsed him he said he would stort to considr my writen work insted of spelings."

This letter, incidentally, was very much more neatly written in the earlier stages than in the later ones.

When Phyllis came to see me at the age of eighteen I gave her the Advanced Matrices test, where her score put her in about the top 15% of the *university* population —a remarkable achievement.

Her attempts at "O" and "A" level were not uniformly successful. At one stage she wrote to me saying she had "a grade 2 pass in Bylogy" (sic), but had failed in Physics and English. "I was dissopinted with my Physics but fortuntly I hove been allowed to continue with Physics 'A' leval without the "O" leval. I am also doing chemestry and Bylogy at 'A' leval."

Later she wrote:

"Dear Proffessor Miles

"I am sarry I hove not writen erler but I was hoping to hove some difinet news for you about what I will be doeing in October but as thing go I am still waiting to here.

"My 'A' leval Results are Biology A Physis A, chemesty D. The only problem is that the univisty are all ful or over full . . . he could fill his next year course with People with good grades now but the univirsty will hove to deside an thes at the end of September."

Finally she was offered a place at a university medical school. On a recent Christmas card she wrote: "Medicen is great fun and not too hard. I hove managed well this tearm."

I do not think any further comment about Phyllis is needed, except to say that even those who are quite severely handicapped, as she was, can still be successful. Suitable teaching and sympathetic encouragement are, of course, essential, and it is important that *all* those who come into contact with a dyslexic child should be aware of the curious nature of the handicap. Once it is recognized, however, I am sure there are grounds for optimism. I do not wish to minimize the difficulties which confront those with dyslexia both in childhood and later, but I hope that the brief sketches in this chapter are sufficient to show the remarkable extent to which these difficulties can be overcome.

Tests of Intelligence, Reading and Spelling

THE following are details of the tests mentioned in the main text (see especially parts of Chapter 1 and pp. 55 *seq.*). No attempt has been made to provide a complete list of the many tests of intelligence, reading and spelling now available, but the present selection includes most of the better known ones.

INTELLIGENCE TESTS:

Advanced Progressive Matrices, Raven, J. C. (H. K. Lewis, 1965)

The Stanford-Binet Intelligence Scale, 3rd revision, Form L-M, Terman, L. M. and Merrill, M. A. (Harrap, 1961)

The Wechsler Intelligence Scale for Children, Wechsler, D. (The Psychological Corporation, 1949)

READING TESTS:

"R.1. Graded Word Reading Test." See *The Psychology and Teaching of Reading*, Schonell, F. J. (Oliver and Boyd, 1951)

The Neale Analysis of Reading Ability, Neale, M. D. (Macmillan, 1966)

The Standard Reading Tests, Daniels, J. C. and Diack, H. (Chatto and Windus, 1958). This book also contains other tests, e.g. of copying, visual discrimination, etc., which may be of use for diagnostic purposes. A variety of language skills are also tested by the *Illinois Test of Psycholinguistic Abilities*, Illinois, 1969

The Holburn Reading Scale (A. F. Watts, 1948) is unsuitable for dyslexic children, since the method of scoring puts a special premium on accuracy, and the result is therefore likely to be artificially low.

SPELLING TESTS:

Graded Spelling Test (suitable for younger children). See *The Standard Reading Tests*, Daniels, J. C. and Diack, H. (details given above)

S.1. Graded Word Spelling Test. See *Diagnostic and Attainment Testing*, Schonell, F. J. (Oliver and Boyd, 1951)

Recognizing the Dyslexic Child
(Notes for Parents and Teachers)

A word of encouragement

Dyslexia is certainly a tiresome handicap but it need not be a major tragedy. The important thing in the first place is that the handicap should be recognized. If parents and teachers understand just what it is that a dyslexic child finds difficult they can help enormously, not only by showing sympathy and giving encouragement but in particular by arranging for suitable teaching.

Does the cap fit?

A dyslexic child differs from other children of the same age in a number of ways. These differences are not shown by all dyslexic children and they occur in a number of different combinations. The seriousness of the difficulties also varies greatly. Parents and teachers may be helped to recognize when the difficulties are due to dyslexia by asking themselves the questions which follow.

* This Appendix has been published as a separate booklet by the Dyslexia Institute. Copies are obtainable from *The Dyslexia Institute, 133 Gresham Road, Staines, Middlesex.* I am grateful to Dr. A. White Franklin, Mr. G. W. S. Gray, and Mrs. S. Naidoo for their help with its preparation.

If the answer to several of the following questions is *Yes*, it is quite possible that your child is appreciably handicapped by dyslexia; and in that case the *Do's* and *Don'ts* mentioned below may be of help to you. ("Several" means perhaps three or four from each section.)

So ask yourself:

(If he* is aged about 8½ or under)

1. Is he still having particular difficulty with **reading**?
2. Is he still having particular difficulty with **spelling**?
3. Does this *surprise* you?
4. Do you get the impression that in matters not connected with reading and spelling he is alert and bright?
5. Does he put figures the wrong way round, e.g. 15 for 51 or ⅽ for 5?
6. Does he put other things the wrong way round, e.g. b and d?
7. In calculations does he need to use bricks or his fingers or marks on paper to help him?
8. Does he have unusual difficulty in remembering arithmetical tables?
9. Was he late in speaking?
10. Is he unusually clumsy?†

(If he is aged 8½ to 12)

11. Does he still make apparently "careless" mistakes in reading?

---

* For "he," read "he or she" throughout. Dyslexia appears to be somewhat more common in boys, but it can perfectly well occur in girls too.

† Some dyslexic children show clumsiness, but by no means all of them.

12. Does he still make strange spelling mistakes?
13. Does he sometimes leave letters out of a word?
14. Does he sometimes put letters in the wrong order?
15. Is he still unsure, sometimes, of the difference between left and right?
16. Are there still occasional b-d confusions?
17. Does he still find arithmetical tables difficult?
18. Does he still need to use his fingers, his toes, or special marks on paper as an aid to calculation?
19. Is it difficult for him to remember the months of the year in correct order?
20. Give him a string of three digits, e.g. 5-2-7, spoken at one second intervals, and ask him to say them in reverse order. The right answer is 7-2-5; does he ever make a mistake, hesitate or become confused?

(If he is aged 12 or over)
21. Are there still occasional inaccuracies in reading?
22. Is his spelling still somewhat odd looking?
23. Do instructions, telephone numbers, etc. sometimes have to be repeated?
24. Does he get "tied up" in saying long words? (Try him with e.g. *preliminary, philosophical, statistical.*)
25. Is he sometimes confused over times and dates?
26. Is a lot of checking needed before he can copy things accurately?
27. Does he still have difficulty with the harder arithmetical tables?
28. In reciting arithmetical tables in the traditional way ("one seven is seven, two sevens are fourteen," etc.)

does he "lose his place," "skip" some of the numbers, or forget what point he has reached?

29. Present him with digits (as in 20 above) but this time give him four digits to say in reverse order, e.g. 4-9-5-8. If he is asked to say them backwards, does he ever make a mistake?

30. Does he slip back to some of his earlier habits when he is tired?

(At all ages)

31. Is there anyone else in his family who has had similar difficulties?

32. Do you have the impression that there are anomalies and inconsistencies in his performance, that he is bright in some ways but seems to have a complete or partial "block" in others of an apparently inexplicable sort?

If for most of these questions you feel the answer is "not particularly" then he is probably not dyslexic. If however, you feel that some of these descriptions "fit" him then it is quite likely that he is dyslexic.

If he is dyslexic, here are some *Do's* and *Don'ts* which may be of help:

1. *Don't* simply brand him as lazy or careless.

2. *Don't* make invidious comparisons with others in his family or with others in his class at school.

3. *Don't* put pressure on him in such a way that he becomes frightened of failing or of letting you down.

4. *Don't*, without his consent, expect him to read out loud to others.

5. *Don't* expect him to learn the spelling of a word by writing it out a few times in the hope that he will remember it; he almost certainly won't!

6. *Don't* be surprised if he tires easily or becomes discouraged.

7. *Don't* be surprised if his handwriting is untidy and irregular; writing is very hard work for him.

8. *Don't* be surprised if his performance is incongruous, that is, if he manages all right on one occasion and not on another.

9. *Don't* just tell him to "try harder."

10. *Do* encourage him in the things that he can do well.

11. *Do* read aloud to him.

12. *Do* express appreciation of effort (e.g. commend him for attempting to write a story and, even if he has made many spelling mistakes, remind him that he has spelled plenty of the words *right*).

13. *Do* encourage him to look at words in detail, a few letters at a time.

14. *Do* discuss frankly with him the things which he finds difficult.

15. *Do* help him to recognize that there are plenty of things which he can do well.

16. *Do* encourage him to go slowly and to take his time.

17. (Most important) *Do* arrange special teaching for him (if possible on a one-to-one basis) by someone who knows about dyslexia.

Schools

If your child is at day-school, have a word with the headmaster, so that between you you can make sure that special individual teaching is given by a suitably informed and sympathetic teacher.

If you are interested in the possibility of boarding school, you may like to know that schools now exist which are organized to deal with the special problems of the dyslexic child. The Dyslexia Institute, 133 Gresham Road, Staines, Middlesex, has a list of private secondary schools which accept children with reading and writing difficulties. You are strongly advised, however, to check *in detail* with the headmasters concerned that the school is suitable for your particular child.

Examinations

If he is entering for an examination, make sure that a certificate saying that he is dyslexic is sent to the examining board. This is normally arranged through the school.

Further enquiries

If you have further enquiries, write to either (*a*) The Dyslexia Institute, 133 Gresham Road, Staines, Middlesex or (*b*) The British Dyslexia Association, 18 The Circus, Bath. Where this is possible, you should ask to be put in touch with your local Dyslexia Association.

Glossary

APHASIA   A condition caused by brain injury (usually as a result of an accident or a stroke) and involving disorders of thought and speech, for example the inability to "find" the word which one wants to say.

AUTISM   A condition in which the sufferer appears to have lost contact with reality and is absorbed in fantasy.

E.E.G. (ELECTROENCEPHALOGRAM) A device which involves the placing of electrodes on the skull and by means of which the rhythms of the brain are recorded.

I.Q. (INTELLIGENCE QUOTIENT) A figure based on the results of a variety of tests of reasoning, etc. A child who obtains a score that is exactly average for his age is said to have an I.Q. of 100. About 16% of children of a given age-group are expected to have an I.Q. of over 115, and about $2\frac{1}{2}$% are expected to have an I.Q. of over 130.

MONOZYGOTIC   Produced by a single zygote (a zygote being the result of the union of a sperm cell from the father and an egg cell from the mother). Monozygotic (or "identical") twins are twins born from a single zygote;

and they thus have basically the same hereditary make-up. In contrast are "dizygotic" (or "fraternal") twins, whose heredity is no more alike than that of ordinary brothers and sisters.

READING AGE   A figure based on the child's performance on a reading test. For example, to say that a child has a reading age of $8\frac{1}{2}$ implies that his attainment at reading is at the level of the average child aged $8\frac{1}{2}$.

SPELLING AGE   A similar figure can be obtained on the basis of a child's performance on a spelling test.

N.B. It is essential to remember with dyslexic children that one must expect a somewhat *irregular* performance in tests of intelligence, reading and spelling. It is therefore more important to observe their behaviour in detail than to be over-concerned with "scoring" it.

Further Reading

FOR those who wish to learn more about dyslexia, the following books are specially recommended:

1. Critchley, M., *The Dyslexic Child* (Heinemann Medical Books, 1971)
2. Franklin, Alfred White, and Naidoo, Sandhya (eds.), *Assessment and Teaching of Dyslexic Children* (Invalid Children's Aid Association, London, 1970)
3. Gillingham, Anna, and Stillman, Bessie W., *Remedial Training for Children with Specific Disability in Reading, Spelling and Penmanship* (Cambridge, Massachusetts, 1956)
4. Hartstein, J. (ed.), *Current Concepts in Dyslexia* (St. Louis, U.S.A., 1973)
5. Hermann, K., *Reading Disability* (Munksgaard, Copenhagen, 1959)
6. Hinshelwood, J., *Letter-, Word-, and Mind-Blindness* (H. K. Lewis, 1900)
7. Hinshelwood, J., *Congenital Word-Blindness* (H. K. Lewis, 1917)
8. Jordan, Dale R., *Dyslexia in the Classroom* (C. E. Merrill Publishing Co., Columbus, Ohio)
9. Klasen, Edith, *The Syndrome of Specific Dyslexia* (Medical Technical Publication Co., Lancaster)

10. MacMeeken, M., *Ocular Dominance in Relation to Development Aphasia* (Ross Foundation, University of London Press, 1939)
11. Miles, T. R., *On Helping the Dyslexic Child* (Methuen Educational, 1970)
12. Miles, T. R., and Miles, E., *More Help for Dyslexic Children* (Methuen Educational, at press)
13. Naidoo, S., *Specific Dyslexia* (Pitman, 1970)
14. Newton, M., *Dyslexia. A Guide for Teachers and Parents* (University of Aston, 1971)
15. Orton, S. T., *Reading, Writing and Speech Problems in Children* (Chapman and Hall, 1937)
16. Vernon, M. D., *Reading and Its Difficulties* (Cambridge University Press, 1972)
17. Zangwill, O. L., *Cerebral Dominance and Its Relation to Psychological Function* (Oliver & Boyd, 1960)

Readers may also like to subscribe to the *Dyslexia Bulletin,* obtainable from The Dyslexia Institute, 133 Gresham Road, Staines, Middlesex, and to the Orton Society, Box 153, Pomfret, Connecticut 06258, U.S.A.

Latest information: the booklet, *People with Dyslexia,* the report of a working party commissioned by the British Council for the Rehabilitation of the Disabled, is not generally available.

Copies may be obtained from: British Council for the Rehabilitation of the Disabled, Tavistock House (South), Tavistock Square, London WC1H 9LB.

Index of Subjects

(Heavy type indicates the main area where a particular topic is discussed)

Index of Names